LIVING WELL WITH
HYPOTHYROIDISM

LIVING WELL WITH
HYPOTHYROIDISM

WHAT YOUR DOCTOR DOESN'T TELL YOU... THAT YOU NEED TO KNOW

MARY J. SHOMON

AN AVON BOOK

Neither the publisher; nor the author; nor any of the medical, health, or wellness practitioners, or thyroid patients quoted in this book takes responsibility for any possible consequences from any treatment, procedure, exercise, dietary modification, action, or application of medication or preparation by any person reading or following the information in this book. The publication of this book does not constitute the practice of medicine, and this book does not attempt to replace your physician or your pharmacist. Before undertaking any course of treatment, the author and publisher advise you to consult with your physician or health practitioner regarding any prescription drugs, vitamins, minerals and food supplements, or other treatments and therapies that would be beneficial for your particular health problems and the dosages that would be best for you.

AVON BOOKS, INC.
An Imprint of HarperCollins*Publishers*
10 East 53rd Street
New York, New York 10022-5299

Copyright © 2000 by Mary J. Shomon
Inside back cover author photograph © David Deal
Interior design by Kellan Peck
Published by arrangement with the author
ISBN: 0-380-80898-6
www.harpercollins.com

Library of Congress Cataloging in Publication Data:
Shomon, Mary J.
    Living well with hypothyroidism : what your doctor doesn't tell you—that you need to know / Mary J. Shomon.
        p.cm.
    "An Avon book."
    Includes bibliographical references and index.
    1. Hypothyroidism—Popular works. I. Title.
RC657.S56 2000
616.4'44—dc21   99-052974

First WholeCare Printing: March 2000

WHOLECARE TRADEMARK REG. U.S. PAT. OFF. AND IN OTHER COUNTRIES, MARCA REGISTRADA, HECHO EN U.S.A.

Printed in the U.S.A.

OPM   10   9   8   7   6   5

For Julia, the future

Nothing will ever be attempted if all possible objections must first be overcome.

SAMUEL JOHNSON

Action is the antidote to despair.

JOAN BAEZ

It is not because things are difficult that we do not dare, it is because we do not dare that they are difficult.

SENECA

ACKNOWLEDGMENTS

I would like to thank my husband and contributing editor, Jon Mathis, for his total dedication to this book and our daughter, his good advice, his excellent brainstorming, his moral support, his backrubs after long days at the computer, and his love. I couldn't have done it without you, BBHBD.

I am very grateful to my agent, Howard Yoon, who spent a tremendous amount of time and fruitful effort helping to make this book a reality. And many thanks to Sarah Durand and Ann McKay Thoroman, my editors, who by intuitively recognizing the need for this book, and others like it, are advancing the mission of patient empowerment.

Much credit goes to John Lowe, D.C., and Kenneth Blanchard, M.D., who spent a great deal of time and energy sharing information with me on their groundbreaking work. They truly believe that people with hypothyroidism deserve the best possible treatments and solutions. They both are the kind of caring, smart doctors we all deserve.

I must also thank my personal physician and friend, Kate Lemmerman, M.D., who in addition to reviewing and making excellent contributions to this book, always amazes me with her open mind, caring spirit, medical talent, and her unique way with an acupuncture needle.

Thanks also to Susan Osborne, D.O., and Zafirah Ahmed, N.D., who are out there every day, fighting the good fight, and looking for real solutions for their patients, and who cared enough to share their thoughts and information with me.

I am indebted to Sandy Levy, Dr. Mike Fitzpatrick, Kelly Cherkes, Dana Godbout Laake, Swami Rameshwarananda, Cynthia White, David Elfstrom, Marge Tolchin, Mindy Green, Pat Rackowski, Larry Ladd, and Ric Blake, who generously shared their thoughts, information, and research findings on behalf of thyroid patients.

Kudos go to Arthur Prange, Robertas Bunevicius, and the rest of the researchers who had the guts to buck the establishment and publish their study on T3 in 1999.

I don't want to forget the supportive and wonderful regulars at the Thyroid Bulletin Board, *http://www.delphi.com/ab-thyroid*, and to my friends at alt.support.thyroid. I also must thank About.com, which has been so supportive of the Thyroid Disease Web site and committed to making my information available worldwide to people with thyroid disease.

To my many friends, "in real life" and online, thanks to you all for bringing me encouragement and joy by phone and email while I was glued to my computer writing this book.

For my parents, Pat and Dan Shomon, I offer thanks for their support, faith, encouragement, love—and delightful pool!

And finally, I am forever grateful to the many hundreds of people with hypothyroidism who took the time to contact me and share their wrenching, hilarious, tragic, infuriating, frightening, empowering—but always honest and heartfelt—stories for this book. While there wasn't space to include every word of every story, everyone who wrote left his or her mark on the project and contributed an amazing amount of spirit, courage, energy, and passion to the book. I wrote this book *for* you, and I couldn't have written it *without* you. May you all live well!

CONTENTS

LIVING WELL WITH
HYPOTHYROIDISM

Introduction

He who enjoys good health is rich, though he knows it not.
ITALIAN PROVERB

Millions of Americans like you wake up each day with hypothyroidism, a disease you don't even know you have. You're fatigued, your hair is falling out, you're gaining weight and depressed. You don't even think to mention your symptoms to the doctor because you assume age, not enough sleep, or too little exercise are to blame. Unfortunately, you don't recognize these problems as common symptoms of hypothyroidism, a condition that affects an estimated 13 million Americans. If you're a woman, you're up against a one-in-eight chance of developing a thyroid disorder during your lifetime. *When you're living with undiagnosed hypothyroidism, you aren't living well.*

Those of you who do mention your problems to the doctor may have a different experience. After reciting a list of symptoms right out of the Thyroid 101 textbook, you are told by your doctor that you are suffering from depression, stress, PMS, menopause, old age, or, simply, that it's probably just "in your head." *If you're living with hypothyroidism and you've been misdiagnosed, that's not living well.*

Countless numbers of you are living unknowingly with hypothyroidism after treatments that your doctors already know can *cause* hypothyroidism. Some doctors actually forget to tell you that after you've had all or part of your thyroid removed due to Graves' disease, nodules, or cancer, you will almost certainly need thyroid hormone replacement. If you've had radioactive iodine treatments or took antithyroid drugs to "kill" your overactive thyroid, your doctor may have forgotten to mention that hypothyroidism is often a result. *Living with an underactive or missing thyroid and the resulting hypothyroidism is not living well.*

Some of you suspect—often correctly—that you are hypothyroid, but you cannot get diagnosed. You have a long list of symptoms and a family history of thyroid problems, but you still can't even get a thyroid test. Sometimes your doctor is arrogant, sometimes ignorant; sometimes you come up against the self-interest that values profit over medical tests. Whatever the reason, doctors repeatedly refuse to test you in the face of symptoms and history. Some of you manage to get tested, only to be told that you're normal by doctors who believe that thyroid-stimulating hormone (TSH) test numbers don't lie—but patients, symptoms, history, and experience do. Your doctors rely on numbers on a page—ignoring common sense, direct examination, and overwhelming symptoms. *When you are living with undiagnosed and untreated hypothyroidism, it's impossible to live well.*

Once you are diagnosed with hypothyroidism, many of you—perhaps even a majority—do not feel well on the standard therapy. One Thyroid Foundation of America study found that up to two-thirds of hypothyroid patients still suffered symptoms—such as muscle pain, lethargy, weight gain, and depression—despite what doctors considered sufficient treatment. If my email inbox is any indication, there are many of you with the same complaints. You're hypothyroid, you don't feel well, and your doctors say, "you're fine, there isn't anything else we can do for you." *Insufficient treatment that leaves you symptomatic is definitely not living well.*

Little helpful information is available. The doctors, the other books about thyroid disease, the pharmaceutical company "educational brochures" and awareness programs, the thyroid patient foundations—they've all closed ranks and usually spout a standard party line: "Take your thyroid pill until your thyroid is in normal range, come back every year for a TSH test, and you're fine." The understanding is, you've got the condition, no point worrying how you got it, how to keep it from getting worse, or whether or not you actually feel well on the standard treatment. If you now have hair loss, depression, fatigue, weight gain, low libido, high cholesterol, or any of dozens of other unresolved symptoms that drastically affect your quality of life—symptoms you never had before your thyroid went bad—hey, what does *that* have to do with anything? You're probably lazy, eating too much, stressed out, not getting enough sleep, not getting enough exercise, getting older, have PMS, or are just plain old depressed. *Just live with it. Live with your hypothyroidism. This is not living well.*

Then there are those of you with special circumstances of hypothyroidism. If you have a baby born with congenital hypothyroidism or a child who has become hypothyroid, you're given a prescription and sent on your way. You need information to ensure that your children *thrive* despite a disease than can profoundly affect their physical and intellectual development. As for thyroid cancer survivors who are hypothyroid due to thyroid cancer surgery, you face the special challenge of periodically going off thyroid hormone completely, allowing yourselves to become extremely hypothyroid, in order to ensure the accuracy of scans to detect cancer recurrence. Doctors provide little or no guidance, expecting that you will just accept living with the hypothyroidism. But there are ways to cope more effectively, to live as well as possible when going hypothyroid prior to a scan. *It's a lack of information that prevents you from living well.*

There are those of you who dare to ask questions. "Is there any thyroid hormone replacement besides levothyroxine?" "Is this really the best dose for me?" "What about the other drugs?" "How about alternative medicine?" You might be ignored, laughed at, patronized, or even in some cases dismissed as a patient. The consensus is that everything to be known is known, and there are no more questions to be asked, especially by patients. Interestingly, new research shows that what have until recently been considered the "standard" treatments don't work as well as so-called "alternative" treatments. Instead of adopting better treatments, many doctors prefer to sit back and call for more studies, while patients suffer needlessly. You're expected to live with your hypothyroidism and not ask questions, quietly enduring. *Living a lifetime of silence,*

*with your valid questions and health concerns unanswered, is not
living well.*

Then, there's the future. What should we know—but don't—
about diagnosing and treating hypothyroidism? What research is
needed, who is looking at possible means of cure or remission,
alternative drugs, and reevaluating optimum thyroid test values?
What are some of the promising treatments that have yet to be
formally studied? *These are questions that need to be answered—
and must be investigated—if any of us is going to live well.*

Millions of people in the U.S. know that it's not enough to just
live *with* hypothyroidism. It's time someone speaks up about how
to live *well* with hypothyroidism.

DO YOU NEED THIS BOOK?

Thirteen million Americans alone have some form of thyroid disease. Almost all forms of thyroid disease lead to a single outcome:
the condition of hypothyroidism—insufficiency of thyroid hormone
due to an underactive, underfunctioning, nonfunctioning, partially
removed, or fully removed thyroid. Whether you have Graves' disease, hyperthyroidism, nodules, a goiter, Hashimoto's autoimmune
thyroid disease, or even thyroid cancer—the result for most of you
is hypothyroidism.

This book is for you if:

- You strongly suspect you have thyroid disease but are having
  difficulty getting a diagnosis by conventional means.
- You aren't sure if your various symptoms point to hypothyroidism, but you're trying to find out more.
- You've been diagnosed with hypothyroidism, told to take this
  pill and come back in a year, and want more information about
  how to live as well as possible with your hypothyroidism.
- You are receiving what your doctor feels is sufficient treatment
  for your hypothyroidism, and you still don't feel well.
- You're an open-minded health practitioner looking for innovative ways to understand and help your hypothyroid patients.

Above all, this book is for you if you want to learn about living well with hypothyroidism from the perspective of empowered patients and caring practitioners.

ABOUT THIS BOOK

Living Well with Hypothyroidism is different. This is *your* book, written *by* a thyroid patient *for* other patients who are going through the familiar ups and downs of diagnosis and treatment. *Living Well with Hypothyroidism* provides the information about hypothyroidism you probably won't find out from your doctor, pharmaceutical companies, patient organizations, or in other books about thyroid disease. I talk honestly, and without allegiance to any pharmaceutical companies or medical organizations, about the risks and symptoms of hypothyroidism, how to truly get a diagnosis, and the many treatments—conventional *and* alternative—to treat the condition and its unresolved symptoms. Ultimately, the book is about living well with hypothyroidism, having the knowledge, tools, and team of health practitioners who can ensure that you feel the best you possibly can.

In this book, you'll find out what your doctor won't tell you about risks, diagnosis, drugs, and alternative and conventional things that work—and don't work—to treat hypothyroidism and its symptoms. You'll also hear the voices of patients, real people who have struggled for diagnosis, learned to deal with doctors, tried different medicines, suffered setbacks, and enjoyed successes. Each person quoted in this book was determined to share his or her own story, ideas, humor, sympathy, hope, advice, and pain with you. I know you will recognize your own experiences, fears and emotions, and be touched and moved by the incredibly honest and poignant stories from patients throughout the world. Above all, you'll know you are not alone.

MY DISCLAIMER

I hope that what you learn in this book will help you decide what questions to ask, or what kinds of doctors to seek, or what types of therapies you might want to pursue. Although I research this subject every day, I don't try to be my own doctor or health practitioner. I ask questions, seek out caring, informed health care providers, and we work in partnership. I don't try to do it myself. Neither should you. So go find the conventional, alternative, complementary, or other practitioners to be your partners in wellness. And don't forget to show them this book.

MY HYPOTHYROIDISM STORY

Before I go any further, I think it might be useful to explain how I got interested in hypothyroidism. First, as I mentioned before, I'm not a doctor. I'm not a health professional. I have an international business degree from Georgetown University. I'm a writer and self-employed strategic communications consultant. Somehow, along the way, my own battle with hypothyroidism led me to manage a popular, patient-oriented Web site on thyroid disease and to launch the only monthly report on conventional and alternative thyroid-related health news and treatments.

Looking back, I'm fairly sure the onset of my thyroid problem occured in early 1993, when I was thirty-two. As a teen and through my twenties, I never had a problem with weight gain. I ate what I wanted, and if I gained a few pounds, I lost it without much difficulty. I joke that in the "old days" all I had to do was cut out a package of chips with lunch every couple of days, switch to diet soda for a week or two, and I'd drop five pounds. I didn't exercise. I worked like a crazy person. I ate terribly. I also smoked a pack and a half of cigarettes a day for more than ten years.

I had about a ten pound weight gain from age thirty to thirty-two, I grew from a size 6/8, to a size 8/10, but didn't worry much about it. Then in the winter of 1993, I published my first book. I was working an intense fulltime job, then coming home and working late into the night on the new book. I had a new boyfriend. It was a period of several months of intense work/book/life excitement and stress, coupled with too little sleep, poor eating habits, and lots of cigarettes and caffeine. I ended up with the worst bronchial infection I'd ever had, which turned into a case of Epstein-Barr so debilitating that I couldn't drag myself out of bed, couldn't go to work for a month, and was so foggy and depressed that I couldn't imagine ever feeling well enough to think clearly, much less return to work. I seriously wondered how I would even muster enough coherence to write a simple memo. I didn't have my thyroid tested at the time, but after looking at my symptoms, and talking to many others who describe similar health crises and resulting brain fog and depression, I believe this is when my thyroid problem started.

A year later—recuperated for the most part but still feeling tired—I started a slow but steady weight gain. I became engaged to my boyfriend in July 1994, and stopped smoking in September of that year. Then the weight gain escalated. I gained 15 pounds between September and my wedding in January 1995, despite an extremely low fat diet, and thirty to forty-five minutes of exercise every night. I was a size 14/16 on my wedding day.

Disgusted with the weight gain and feeling increasingly depressed, I started smoking again. No weight lost, none gained, and I was still depressed. At that point, I felt dumpy, overweight, depressed, and then six months later, in July 1995, I started having trouble getting a full breath. The doctor thought I had developed asthma. At that point, I quit smoking—for good—and a few more pounds piled on. A month after I quit, the doctor decided to run some blood tests because I was again complaining that I didn't feel well. The doctor called a few days later and said that I had "low thyroid," and she'd called in a prescription for me. She put me on Thyrolar™ and said to come in about six weeks later for a checkup. I had absolutely no idea what a thyroid was or even where it was located.

After I was diagnosed, I continued developing all kinds of symptoms that mystified my doctor and me. My eyes were dry and gritty and my menstrual periods became heavier and more frequent. My skin started flaking. I had headaches. I asked if it could be the thyroid problem. My doctor wasn't sure about a direct connection, and sent me for second opinions from an infectious disease specialist, a pulmonary specialist, and an internist. I had an MRI. I had a consultation with an endocrinologist, who acknowledged that some of the symptoms I had probably *were* due to my thyroid. She ran an antibodies test—at my request—but said it wasn't necessary because it didn't matter *why* I was hypothyroid. I just was. The test revealed the antibodies that signal Hashimoto's disease. I asked what that meant, and the endocrinologist said it didn't change the treatment, so I didn't have to worry about it.

The endocrinologist said it was just coincidence that I was a size 8 who could eat anything I wanted before my thyroid went bad, and that less than a year later, I was a size 12 battling an extra thirty pounds and barely staving off additional gain on even the most rigorous adherence to Weight Watchers™. She suggested that the other symptoms would eventually relax. The way she put it was:

> In four months or so, you'll look back and realize how much better you feel than you do now. It's going to be relative, and so gradual that it won't be dramatic. One day down the road, you'll just realize you feel better than you do now.

So I waited my four months. And I still didn't feel quite well. Far better than before, yes, but still not right. So I read, and I read. And then I got a computer, and I surfed the Web. I started to disseminate information I found via the online Usenet newsgroup alt.support.thyroid, and talk with other thyroid patients. And I found out that hair falling out, weird periods, difficulty losing weight, carpal tunnel syndrome, and depression were all utterly "normal" symptoms of hypothyroidism. Maybe some of the information wasn't what I *wanted* to hear, but I *needed* to hear it!

It was a revelation. Knowing what was and wasn't related to my thyroid was far better than not knowing. There were times I felt so sick that I secretly worried I had some incurable disease that the doctors had overlooked. Realizing that symptoms were related to the thyroid also gave me something to shoot for—fixing my thyroid—instead of running around taking pill after pill or visiting high-priced specialists for every supposedly new, but actually thyroid-related, symptom that appeared.

Later, I assembled a lot of my information and created a thyroid disease Web site—http://thyroid.about.com—at the popular search engine/community portal site About.com (which was known as the Mining Company when I first started my site.) At the site,

I offer dozens of articles on thyroid disease, maintain an active bulletin board, and provide links to hundreds of online sources of conventional and alternative thyroid information. Back in July 1997, I also started a separate newsletter called *Sticking Out Our Necks* that offers the latest thyroid-related news on health, drugs, treatments, tests, companies, and alternative therapies for hypothyroidism and its symptoms. I've also recently expanded the newsletter to a printed version by regular mail.

Two years ago, I assembled the hundreds of doctor recommendations I've received and created what is known as the *Thyroid Top Doc Directory*, a state-by-state and international listing of the best doctors recommended by thyroid patients around the world. And along the way, despite my hypothyroidism, I even succeeded at my most important project of all, giving birth to my wonderful daughter, Julia, in late 1997.

Every day for the past five years I've studied as much as I can about thyroid disease and hypothyroidism, searched for information on conventional and alternative ways to diagnose and treat hypothyroidism, and turned around and put that information out via my Web page and my news report. As part of my educational mission, I've answered thousands of emails from people with hypothyroidism from the U.S., Canada, England, Germany, Australia, Indonesia, Saudi Arabia, Pakistan, Brazil, seemingly everywhere. Over and over again, people write, pouring out their hearts, sharing the same concerns, the same problems:

> For five years, I suffered from increasingly debilitating symptoms, and no doctors ever correlated my list of symptoms as clear evidence of hypothyroidism. I was always feeling cold, I had unending fatigue, sometimes sleeping eighteen to twenty hours a night on weekends and twelve hours a night during the week, low blood pressure, allergy and sinus problems, bone and joint pain, depression, memory loss, a very sleepy state I now call brain fog, depression, and mood swings. You'd be moody too if you were constantly exhausted and often confused and overwhelmed by things that used to be crystal clear to you. In five years, I slowly evolved from a highly productive, very social, and caring person to someone who chose to be alone and felt like a failure in life. I was self-isolated—secretly feared that I had early

Alzheimer's, or worse, undiagnosed cancer or another major
illness . . .

Alice

At the age of thirty, I thought I was dying inside. My cholesterol was
436. My doctor called me and asked, "What do you eat?" I told him
I didn't eat that badly. He ran more tests and I asked him to check
my thyroid. He said, "Okay but I don't think that's it." Well it was.
My TSH was 218! He said I should be in a coma.

Tracy

My family doctor referred me a specialist, head of endocrinology
department, suspecting hypothyroidism. I saw the specialist, complaining of my symptoms, including disgusting weight gain, depression, and lack of energy. He laughed at me and said that I was
pregnant. I said, "No, I'm not . . . positively without a doubt I am
not pregnant." He kept laughing, and said, "Yes you are, I'll see you
in nine months!" And he walked out of the room. That's it. I was in
tears and angry when I left. I went the next day to my gynecologist's
office, where a pregnancy blood test proved that I was *not* pregnant.
I was referred to another doctor, who, based upon my skin, eyes,
blood test, and reflexes, immediately diagnosed me with Hashimoto's
disease. I just want people to believe that they themselves know when
their body is acting crazy. Find a doctor who will help—not think
you are insane or pregnant!

LuAnn

When you receive dozens of emails like this every single day
for years, it's obvious something is wrong, and someone needs to
do something about it. That's why I wrote this book.

ABOUT THE INTERNET

Throughout this book, there are references to Web sites, emails,
and Internet-based resources. If you have access to the Internet,
you can visit this book's Web site, at http://www.thyroid-info.com.
The site features all the Web sites mentioned in the book, orga-

nized as up-to-date links, along with updated information and late-breaking news.

I hope these references don't intimidate those of you who are not veteran Web surfers or who don't consider yourselves computer literate. The reason I wrote this book is that I know that for every email, bulletin board post, or phone call I've received saying: "Help, I feel so alone" or "My doctor won't test me!" or "I'm gaining weight but my TSH is normal!" or "Why won't my doctor even *test* my thyroid?" there are so many more of you out there who are not online who are in this same situation.

There are so many of us, millions actually. And we're finally going to start talking out loud about what many of us have been suffering with alone, silently, for many years.

CHALLENGING THE DOCTRINE, GOING BEYOND THE CONVENTIONAL

In this book, I do a bit of ranting and raving about some doctors, but I don't want you to think that I have a vendetta against the medical establishment. I thank the heavens that there are doctors and practitioners who love medicine, who love the idea of caring for, healing, and curing patients. These wonderful doctors keep asking the right questions, keep looking for better answers, really listen to their patients, and are passionate about finding new ways to be our partners in the search for wellness. I have met many wonderful doctors—including the doctors who have contributed to this book, and the doctors who care for me personally—and they are sympathetic, smart women and men I consider to be my friends, colleagues and partners in wellness. They march to the beat of a different drummer, and think for themselves. I respect them completely.

But unfortunately, all doctors are not like them. Some doctors end up believing that everything there is to be known about diagnosing and treating hypothyroidism is already understood. Scary, isn't it, that some medical professionals—the people we entrust with our lives and our health—can be that narrow-minded?

You'll soon find out that new research is questioning the very validity of the TSH blood test ranges used to diagnose and manage hypothyroidism. Other research has also demonstrated what many thyroid patients, myself included, have known for a long time— that people don't feel as well on levothyroxine (i.e., Synthroid™) alone as they do with the addition of a *second* thyroid hormone. This report was published in the *New England Journal of Medicine*. At the same time, the majority of doctors continue to rely exclusively on the TSH test and levothyroxine, condemning people to undiagnosed or undertreated hypothyroidism, with the resulting mediocre or poor health and diminished quality of life.

One woman with hypothyroidism asked me:

> Why did the doctors stop listening to the patients' valid concerns and start ignoring total deterioration in health in order to devote themselves to the results of a test and treatment with only one drug?

That is an important question, one that I try to answer in this book. The opinions of the mainstream medical establishment are well represented in the other books and patient-oriented pamphlets on thyroid disease, the books and materials that often leave people desperate to feel well again. Now it's time that the millions of patients with hypothyroidism—people who actually have to live with the condition—have a chance to be heard and, ultimately, to live well.

PART I

SIGNS, SYMPTOMS, DIAGNOSIS, AND TREATMENT

CHAPTER 1

What is Hypothyroidism?

*They do certainly give very strange, and newfangled,
names to diseases.*
PLATO

The thyroid is not a particularly well-known or well-understood organ in the body. Some people have a vague idea of the thyroid as something in the neck that, when malfunctioning, makes you gain weight or develop a goiter. That's about all the information many people can muster.

The thyroid gland, however, is an essential organ, governing basic aspects of nearly every facet of your health. In the long term, you can't live without the hormones produced by your thyroid. Those hormones regulate the body's use of energy, an essential function to life and health.

WHAT IS THE THYROID?

The *thyroid gland* is shaped a little like a butterfly, and is located in the lower part of your neck, in front of your windpipe. You'll know generally where the thyroid is located if you think of it as sitting behind the Adam's apple, which usually sticks out farther from a man's neck than from a woman's.

The name "thyroid" comes from the Greek word, *thyreoeides*, meaning "shield-shaped." The two "wings" of the butterfly are known as the *lobes* of the thyroid, and the area connecting the two lobes is known as the *isthmus*. It's a small gland, and normally weighs only about an ounce.

Roughly speaking, a *gland* is a discrete and separate soft body made up of a large number of vessels that produce, store, and release—or secrete—some substance. Your thyroid is one of these glands.

Some glands secrete their products outside the body, some inside. Those that secrete their products on the inside of the body and, more specifically, secrete hormonal and metabolic substances, are known as *endocrine glands*. The thyroid is an endocrine gland, as are the parathyroids, the adrenal gland, the pancreas, and the pituitary gland. Diabetes, like thyroid disease, is considered an endocrine disorder. A doctor who specializes in treating patients with endocrine problems is called an endocrinologist.

Hormones are internal secretions carried in the blood to various organs. The thyroid's main purpose is to produce, store, and release two key thyroid hormones, *triiodothyronine (T3)* and *thyroxine (T4)*. Thyroid cells are the only body cells that are able to absorb *iodine*. The thyroid takes in iodine, obtained through food, iodized salt, or supplements, and combines that iodine with the amino acid *tyrosine*, converting the iodine/tyrosine combination into T3 and T4. The "3" and the "4" refer to the number of iodine molecules in each thyroid hormone molecule. A healthy, functioning thyroid produces about 80 percent T4 and 20 percent T3. T3 is considered the biologically active hormone and is several times stronger than T4.

The T3 and T4 thyroid hormones travel through the bloodstream throughout the body helping cells to convert oxygen and calories into energy. Thyroid hormones control *metabolism*—the process by which oxygen and calories are converted to energy for use by cells and organs. There's not a single cell in your body that doesn't depend on thyroid hormone for regulation and for energy in some form.

The thyroid produces some T3, but the rest of the T3 needed by the body is actually formed from the mostly inactive T4 by the removal of one iodine molecule, a process sometimes referred to as *T4 to T3 conversion*, or by the more scientific term *mono-deiodination*. This conversion of T4 to T3 can take place in some organs other than the thyroid, including the *hypothalamus*, a part of your brain.

Now that you have some idea of what the thyroid is and its location and function, let's look in more detail at how it fits into the overall functioning of the body.

The Thyroid Gland: Setting the Pace

When the thyroid works normally, it produces and secretes the amount of T4 and T3 necessary to keep many bodily functions at their proper pace. However, the thyroid does not do this alone. It works instead as part of a system that also includes the pituitary gland and the hypothalamus. The *pituitary gland* is another endocrine gland, located at the base of your brain.

Here's how the system works. The hypothalamus constantly monitors the pace of many of the body's functions. It also monitors and reacts to a number of other factors, including outside environmental factors such as heat, cold, and stress. If the hypothalamus senses that certain adjustments are needed to react to any of these factors, then it produces *thyrotropin-releasing hormone, (TRH)*.

TRH is sent from the hypothalamus to the pituitary gland. The pituitary gland then produces a substance called *thyrotropin,* which is also known as *thyroid-stimulating hormone (TSH)*. The pituitary gland also monitors the body and can release TSH based on the thyroid hormones in the blood. TSH is sent to the thyroid gland, where it causes production, storage, and release of more T3 and T4.

Released thyroid hormones move into the bloodstream, carried by a plasma protein known as *thyroxine-binding globulin (TBG)*.

Now in the bloodstream, the thyroid hormone travels throughout the body, carrying orders to the various bodily organs. Upon arriving at a particular tissue in the body, thyroid hormones interact with receptors located inside the nucleus of the cells. Interaction of the hormone and the receptor will trigger a certain function, giving directions to that tissue regarding the rate at which it should operate.

When the hypothalamus senses that the need for increased thyroid hormone production has ended, it reduces production of TRH, the pituitary decreases production of TSH, and production of the thyroid hormone, in turn, decreases. By this system, many of the body's organs are kept working at the proper pace.

WHAT IS HYPOTHYROIDISM?

When your thyroid starts producing too much thyroid hormone and the balancing system doesn't function properly, then you become *hyperthyroid*. Your body goes into overdrive, gets sped up, causing an increased heart rate, increased blood pressure, and burning more calories more quickly. Conversely, when the thyroid isn't functioning properly, or part or all of the thyroid has been removed, you don't have enough thyroid hormone, and you become *hypothyroid*. Your body is moving on "slow" speed, with lower heart rate, lower blood pressure, lower body temperature, and you burn fewer calories, more slowly.

Hypothyroidism is not really a disease unto itself, rather it's a condition in which there is insufficient thyroid hormone in the body, and the body therefore requires thyroid hormone replacement. Hypothyroidism can result from autoimmune Hashimoto's disease or nodules or a temporary inflammation of the thyroid, known as thyroiditis. Hashimoto's disease results when antibodies attach themselves to proteins in the thyroid tissue. The attachment process is a declaration of war to the rest of the immune system, and the thyroid is then invaded by immune cells that progressively destroy the hormone-producing thyroid tissue in a misguided effort to fend off the perceived invader.

In some cases, hypothyroidism results from treatment for Graves' disease. Graves' disease is an autoimmune disease in which the thyroid goes into uncontrolled overproduction. Antithyroid drugs or radioactive iodine therapy usually treat Graves' disease. Both treatments partially or fully disable the thyroid's function. Sometimes Graves' disease requires surgical removal of the thyroid.

Some people have had all or part of their thyroids surgically removed as a treatment for thyroid cancer, nodules, goiters, or other thyroid problems, and are now hypothyroid.

Severe deficiency of iodine, and in some cases too much iodine, can cause hypothyroidism. There are some drugs, such as lithium and amiodarone, that cause hypothyroidism. Radiation and cancer treatments to the neck and chest areas can frequently cause hypothyroidism. A comprehensive look at the risk factors and causes of hypothyroidism is included in chapter 2.

HOW IS HYPOTHYROIDISM TRADITIONALLY DIAGNOSED?

Most conventional doctors rely on a test known as the TSH test to diagnose hypothyroidism. The TSH test is the sensitive blood test that measures the amount of thyroid-stimulating hormone—TSH—in your bloodstream. The TSH level remains in the normal range when the thyroid gland is healthy and functioning normally. Elevated TSH is considered indicative of hypothyroidism.

You'll need to know what the normal values are for the lab where your doctor sends your blood because "normal" varies from lab to lab. Typical throughout North America, however, is a "normal" TSH range from about 0.3-0.5 to 4.7-5.5. At the lab where they send my blood, for example, a TSH of over 5.5 is hypothyroid, under 0.5 is hyperthyroid. Anywhere in between is considered "normal."

Values below the lower range can indicate hyperthyroidism, an overactive thyroid. Values above the top range indicate hypothyroidism, an underactive thyroid. The higher the number, the more hypothyroid you are, and therefore the less functional your thyroid is considered to be.

Hyperthyroid ⇦	.3 to .6	TSH "Normal" Range	4.7 to 6	Hypothyroid ⇨
Numbers lower than .3 to .6 are usually considered Hyperthroid (overactive)	Low end of the range (varies lab to lab)	Normal TSH range means that the thyroid is considered "euthyroid," or normal, neither hyperthyroid nor hypothyroid	Top end of the range (varies lab to lab)	Numbers above 4.7 to 6 are usually considered Hypothyroid (underactive)

The idea that *low* TSH means hyperthyroidism/overactive thyroid function, and *high* TSH means hypothyroidism/underactive thyroid can be confusing. Keep in mind, the pituitary gland releases TSH based on the amount of thyroid hormones in the blood. TSH is considered a messenger that says to the thyroid, "produce more hormone." If you already have enough thyroid hormone, or even too much, there's no need for much TSH at all to deliver the "produce more hormone" message. You already have enough hormone, so TSH levels drop, and become *low*, when you're hyperthyroid. Conversely, if you don't have enough thyroid hormone because of an underfunctioning or nonexistent thyroid gland, more TSH will be produced in order to keep telling the thyroid, "produce more hormone." This is why TSH levels are *high* when you're hypothyroid.

This also explains why doctors will cut your dosage if your TSH is too low, and they'll give you more thyroid hormone if your TSH is too high.

TSH tests can be expensive. They can run from $30 to $100 depending on the lab, and even more if there are substantial markups by doctors' offices. Some endocrinologists have expensive analysis machines that can do a TSH test on the premises in a short amount of time, but most doctors send your blood to a lab for testing.

There are new, less expensive "instant" TSH tests now on the market. These tests mainly determine if your TSH is above "normal" range, with no specific assessment of the number itself. In my opinion, these tests might be useful for first-level, broad screening to uncover more serious hypothyroidism in people who otherwise would not be tested at all, but should not be used for monitoring purposes.

Blood Tests for Other Thyroid Levels

Other levels that are sometimes tested along with TSH:

• *Total T4/Total Thyroxine*—Normal range runs from approximately 4.5 to 12.5. A reading of less than 4.5, along with elevated TSH, is considered indicative of hypothyroidism. The combination of low T4 with *low* TSH can indicate a pituitary problem.

• *Free T4/Free Thyroxine*—Normal range is 0.7-2.0 and less than 0.7 is considered indicative of possible hypothyroidism.

• *Total T3*—This test has a normal range of approximately 80 to 220 and less than 80 can be indicative of hypothyroidism.

• *Free T3*—Normal range is approximately 2.3 to 4.2, and less than 2.3 can be indicative of hypothroidism.

Antibodies Tests

Many doctors consider the TSH thyroid panel the only test needed for diagnosis of hypothyroidism. Some doctors, however, will test to determine if you have what are known as "antibodies" or antithyroid antibodies (sometimes abbreviated as ATA). An antibodies test determines whether you have an autoimmune thyroid problem. An autoimmune reaction is when the body acts as if one of its own organs is a foreign substance and tries to "attack" it. When this happens with your thyroid, antibodies are developed against your own thyroid that can either make it less able to function (Hashimoto's hypothyroidism) or send it into hyperfunctioning (Graves' disease/hyperthyroidism). The normal ranges for antibodies seem to vary somewhat at each lab, so be sure to find out what the normal range is for your doctor's lab.

TRH Test

In an article in *Alternative Medicine* magazine, Dr. Rafael Kellman called the TRH (thyrotropin-releasing hormone) stimulation test the "gold standard for accurately detecting an underactive thyroid." In a TRH test, TSH is measured prior to an injection of TRH. About a half-hour later, TSH is measured again. The TRH injection should have stimulated the pituitary gland to secrete TSH. If the pituitary does not secrete TSH at all and TSH does not elevate, then a pituitary abnormality may be investigated, or this may be indicative of hyperthyroidism. If the second TSH level is high, however, the test may point to hypothyroidism. Dr. Kellman feels that a TSH level over ten during a TRH test indicates underactivity or potential hypothyroidism. Some doctors feel the TSH has to rise above 20 or even 30 to indicate hypothyroidism.

Writes Dr. Kellman:

> Of the patients I've seen with three or more typical symptoms of underactive thyroid but who have tested "normal" in standard tests, 35 to 40 percent actually have underactive thyroids based on the TRH test.

Dr. Kellman also believes that the TRH test can uncover the physiological causes behind an underfunctioning thyroid, while the other tests uncover only the underfunction itself.

Reverse T3 Test

When the body is under stress, instead of converting T4 into T3—the active form of thyroid hormone that works at the cellular level—the body makes what is known as Reverse T3 (RT3), an inactive form of the T3 hormone, to conserve energy. Some practitioners believe that even when stress is relieved, in some people the body continues to manufacture RT3 instead of active T3. This in turn creates a thyroid problem at the cellular level, yet the TSH lab values may well be normal. RT3 tests, therefore, have become more popular with open-minded doctors who are looking to assess a person's full range of thyroid function. RT3 can be measured with a blood test.

Basal Body Temperature Test

It's medically known that thyroid hormones have a direct effect on the basal, or resting, metabolic rate. And while hypothermia, or lowered body temperature, is a known and medically accepted symptom of hypothyroidism, the use of body temperature as a diagnostic tool is more controversial. Broda Barnes, M.D., made the public more widely aware of the use of axillary (underarm) basal body temperature (BBT) as a symptom and diagnostic tool for hypothyroidism. It is a diagnostic and monitoring method still used by a variety of complementary and alternative physicians and health care practitioners. It is also the only way to assess metabolic function that is free to the patient.

To measure your own BBT, use an oral glass/Mercury thermometer. Shake the thermometer down before going to bed, and leave it close by and within reach. As soon as you wake up, with a minimum of movement, put the thermometer in your armpit, next to the skin, and leave it in place for ten minutes. Record the readings for three to five consecutive days. Women who still have their menstrual period should not test on the first five days of their period but can begin on day 5. Men, and girls and women who are not menstruating, can test any time of the month.

If the average BBT is below 97.6 Fahrenheit, many complementary practitioners would strongly consider a diagnosis of an underfunctioning thyroid or insufficient thyroid hormone replacement. An average BBT between 97.8 and 98.2 is considered normal. Temperatures from 97.6 to 98.0 degrees Fahrenheit are considered evidence of possible hypothyroidism, and temperatures less than 97.6 degrees can be even more indicative of hypothyroidism. Some practitioners, however, consider any temperature under 98 degrees to be indicative of hypothyroidism.

For patients of Dr. Susan Osborne, an osteopathic physician in Floyd, Virginia, one part of monitoring thyroid function is to involve patients in taking body temperatures and pulse at different times of the day. According to Dr. Osborne:

> We have patients keep a diary of temperatures and pulses. This helps us to diagnose hypothyroidism, and after treatment, to monitor whether too much thyroid medicine might be releasing at particular times of the day. We have patients bring a logbook. These measurements are also free and can be done anytime by the patient.

You don't need to be an expert in thyroid physiology and testing in order to be an advocate for your own health and wellness. But if you're interested in a more detailed explanation of thyroid function physiology, the "Resources" appendix at the back of this book contains a number of books and Web sites that can offer detailed, in-depth information.

CHAPTER 2

Are You at Risk for Hypothyroidism?

A jug fills drop by drop.
BUDDHA

First, let's take a look at the various risk factors for hypothyroidism. Having one, or even many, of these risk factors does not necessarily mean you are or will become hypothyroid. But if you suspect you might be hypothyroid and have not been diagnosed yet, a review of the various factors that put you at risk can be an important diagnostic clue. Or if you *have* been diagnosed and wonder how you became hypothroid, you may find some ideas here.

RISK FACTORS FOR HYPOTHROIDISM

A Family History of Thyroid Problems

If you have a parent, sibling, or child with autoimmune thyroid problems, nodules, or goiters, then you are at greater risk for developing a thyroid problem. Research shows that up to 50 percent of all first-degree relatives of people with autoimmune thyroid disease themselves have thyroid antibodies that may be a marker for later development of clinical autoimmune hypothroidism.

It's likely that someone in your family has a thyroid problem and you don't know about it. He or she just doesn't mention it or is embarrassed to talk about it. For years, thyroid problems have been downplayed, misunderstood, and portrayed as unimportant.

So it's not safe to assume you know about family thyroid problems unless you ask specifically and listen carefully.

If you ask your mother about diseases she's had, thyroid may never be mentioned. But ask about the thyroid specifically, and she might remember an episode of thyroid trouble after a pregnancy. Sometimes, your family member won't even refer to the thyroid. You might hear about a relative who is overweight because "she has a gland problem and has to take medication for it." Or a family member might tell you in passing that "goiters run in the family."

Ask questions. Ask about thyroid, goiters, metabolism, "glandular problems"—all ways people describe thyroid problems. If you suspect you might have thyroid disease, you might need to play detective a bit to get this sort of family history. In the face of a doctor reluctant to test your thyroid, however, a clear family history can be valuable ammunition in your search for a diagnosis.

Researching her family thyroid history, Nancy had this interesting conversation with her parents:

> I was having dinner with my folks, now seventy-five and seventy-six year old, and I was telling them of my week's events with the "Thyroid Adventure." I was asking them if they have ever had any history of thyroid problems. Dad said he just started taking thyroid meds for *hyperthyroid* condition, and Mom said, "Oh yes! My doctor had me on thyroid medication right after you were born in 1949 because I was anemic, but after we moved, which was a year later, I just quit taking it!" Okay, Mom, and you never thought about your low blood pressure, or the fact that you had to take a nap almost daily and that you had an increasing weight gain for the next half century?

Needless to say, Nancy *and* her mother will be getting hypothyroidism treatment from now on.

A Personal History of Thyroid Problems or Irregularities

Having any history of thyroid problems yourself puts you at greater risk for developing hypothyroidism. In some cases, your doctor may have told you that he or she was "monitoring" your thyroid because blood test results were inconclusive or borderline. Your doctor might have diagnosed a goiter or nodule but decided it didn't warrant treatment. Some of you may not even remember the diagnosis, but know that years ago, you took thyroid hormone for a period of time. You may have had a short episode of thyroid trouble after a pregnancy, or after an illness, and may have had a diagnosis of something called "transient"—or temporary—thyroiditis or hypothyroidism. Past thyroid problems increase your chances of later developing hypothyroidism.

Hyperthyroidism Treatment/Thyroid Surgery, Radioactive Iodine (RAI) or Antithyroid Drugs

Amazingly, some doctors do *not* tell their patients that treatments that involve removing or disabling the thyroid can result in hypothyroidism. Some people have all or part of the thyroid surgically removed to treat nodules or Graves' disease. In other cases, thyroid treatment for hyperthyroidism can involve radioactive iodine (RAI) or antithyroid drugs, which make the thyroid either partially or fully inactive.

Some of the literature given to patients overemphasizes the fact that everyone who has RAI does not necessarily become hypothyroid or need thyroid hormone replacement. It's true that some patients do not become hypothyroid after these treatments. In general, however, many do become hypothyroid and will need thyroid hormone replacement to avoid suffering from hypothyroidism symptoms.

If you have had thyroid surgery, RAI, or have taken antithyroid drugs, you should monitor yourself very carefully for the onset of hypothyroidism symptoms. At the same time, you will probably want to have regular TSH blood tests to monitor your thyroid function via your bloodwork as well.

Thyroid Cancer Surgery

When you've had your thyroid removed in part or in full due to thyroid cancer, you will likely be prescribed thyroid hormone for two reasons: to treat the resulting hypothyroidism and to prevent cancer recurrence. Most knowledgeable thyroid cancer experts recommend suppression of TSH into very low ranges as a way to prevent recurrence of the cancer. Patients having a scan to detect any cancer recurrence, however, are often required to go off their thyroid medicine and experience hypothyroid symptoms because an elevated TSH is needed to get an accurate scan.

Pituitary Tumors and Pituitary Disease

Less common, but still a known cause of hypothyroidism, are problems with the pituitary gland, including diseases or tumors that cause pituitary failure and hypothyroidism.

Other Autoimmune or Endocrine Diseases

If you or close family members have other autoimmune or endocrine diseases, you have a slightly increased chance of developing autoimmune thyroid disease. In particular, there are suspected relationships among chronic fatigue immune dysfunction syndrome (also known as CFS or CFIDS), fibromyalgia, and autoimmune thyroid problems. Other diseases that are associated with a slightly increased chance of developing autoimmune thyroid disease include Crohn's disease, Addison's disease, insulin-dependent (type I) diabetes, multiple sclerosis, pernicious anemia, scleroderma, and Sjögren's syndrome.

Epstein-Barr Virus (EBV) and Mononucleosis

While the evidence is mainly anecdotal, some doctors suspect that there may be a relationship between having had Epstein-Barr virus (EBV) and/or mononucleosis, and later developing autoimmune thyroid disease. I had mononucleosis at seventeen and then had a very bad EBV flareup when I was thirty-one. I suspect that the total exhaustion, and nearly two-month recuperation from the EBV, followed by the beginning of weight gain, was likely the onset of the thyroid problems for me. I have received many emails from people who also reported having had teenage cases of mononucleosis, only to have flareups of Epstein-Barr immediately preceding the diagnosis of hypothyroidism in adulthood.

Aging

If you are over sixty, chances are greater that your thyroid may become problematic than for a younger person. According to the American Thyroid Association (ATA), large population studies have shown that as many as one woman in every ten over the age of sixty-five has a blood level of TSH that is above normal, making her hypothyroid. According to the American Medical Women's Association, the elderly are more likely to suffer from hypothyroidism, and by age 60, as many as 17 percent of women have an underactive thyroid. In the ever-confusing world of statistics, the American Association of Clinical Endocrinologists (AACE) states that thyroid problems affect one in eight women ages 35 to 65 and one in five women—20 percent—over 65. Because the symptoms of hypothyroidism can be so similar to those related to aging, it is more difficult for doctors to spot thyroid disease in older patients.

Fertility, Pregnancy, and Hormonal Issues

Being a woman means you are more likely to develop thyroid disease than men. According to the American Medical Women's Association, women are five to eight times more likely than men to suffer from an overactive or underactive thyroid, and approximately one woman in eight will develop a thyroid disorder during her lifetime.

If you have had a baby in the past year, you are at increased risk for a variety of thyroid problems, including a short-term problem known as post-partum thyroiditis. Post-partum is also a time when underlying full-scale thyroid problems become evident and are diagnosed. Some doctors estimate that as many as 5 to 10 percent of women develop a thyroid problem after delivery. Most of these women have never had any thyroid problem in the past. Some doctors are now beginning to test carefully for hypothyroidism, as it often underlies cases of post-partum depression.

While some post-partum cases of hypothyroidism are temporary, the period after pregnancy is also a common time for permanent thyroid problems to surface. Bess was thirty-five and had just had her third child when she was diagnosed with post-partum hypothyroidism:

> At the time, I was still nursing my five-month-old son. Even though he was already taking baby food, he was still getting up in the night for feedings. I was exhausted, depressed, overweight, and looked terrible. My face was puffy and swollen, and I was always cold. I would wake up in the mornings and cry because I did not want to get out of bed. My mother urged me to see a doctor, but I dragged my feet thinking I was just unable to cope with my new infant and other children. I finally saw a doctor. He felt there was "nothing wrong with me that diet and exercise wouldn't help." However, he did run some blood tests. A couple of days later I received a call from my doctor. He needed to see me right away for a consultation in his office. That is when I found out why I was a wreck. He seemed surprised by my lab results, informing me that "I wasn't even on the charts," and that I was about as sick as I could be. Even though he explained what thyroid disease is, he felt confident that I would eventually be fine. . . . Anyway, here I sit taking Synthroid for the "rest of my life." So much for "post-partum."

Unfortunately, not all doctors are aware that there are periods when women are more prone to developing thyroid problems, such as after having a baby. One new mother who wrote to me had a doctor who clearly wasn't very informed:

> When I went to the endocrinologist, he was adamant that I did not have a thyroid problem. His strongest statement was that "if you were hypothyroid, you could never have become pregnant."

Miscarriage is now also being found to be associated in some cases with the presence of thyroid antibodies, high-normal levels of TSH, or underlying and undiagnosed hypothyroidism. The risk of miscarriage is higher when a woman is positive for antithyroid antibodies; some researchers estimate that the risk of miscarriage is twice as high. In addition, they are finding that the presence of antibodies prior to miscarriage may trigger the post-miscarriage onset of thyroid problems.

Menopause

By the end of 1999, an estimated 50 million American women reached menopause, about 18 percent of the total U.S. population. Many of these menopausal women will take hormone replacement therapy, yet an estimated one-third of those women still experience symptoms such as mood swings, depression, and sleep disturbances that are attributed to "menopause" but may in fact be due to undiagnosed thyroid problems. Unfortunately, according to a survey conducted by the American Association of Clinical Endocrinologists, only one in four women who have discussed menopause with their physician received a recommendation to be tested for thyroid disease.

Thyroid problems are known to surface at periods of hormonal upheaval and are more common just prior to or during menopause. As with aging, thyroid problems can be difficult to detect because symptoms are similar to menopause. If you're menopausal and having hormone levels checked, always be sure your doctor includes a thyroid TSH test as well.

Smoking and Smoking Cessation

If you are or were a smoker, you have an increased risk of hypothyroidism. Cigarettes contain thiocyanate, a chemical that adversely affects the thyroid gland and acts as an antithyroid agent. Researchers have found that smoking may increase the risk of hypothyroidism in patients with Hashimoto's thyroiditis.

If you have recently quit smoking, this may also be a time when underlying thyroid disease becomes apparent. Anecdotally, I have also heard from many women who, like me, were diagnosed with thyroid disease soon after they quit smoking. I've even wondered if there is a direct link, but that seems unlikely. More likely, I'd suspect that the nicotine "buzz" from smoking creates an artificially higher metabolism that hides the fatigue and exhaustion and weight gain commonly seen in hypothyroidism. When a smoker with underlying hypothyroidism quits, the full effects of hypothyroidism are felt, and metabolism slows down.

The nonsmoking advocates tell us that the average person gains no more than about four to six pounds after smoking. But hidden thyroid problems may explain why some who quit end up gaining far more than that. (Me, for example!) If you are a smoker with undiagnosed thyroid dysfunction, stopping seems to be a metabolic/ weight gain double whammy, as you lose the appetite suppressant, metabolism-upping effects of nicotine and then experience the full effects of the hypothyroidism.

Of course, this is *not* a reason not to quit! You're still better off not smoking and gaining some weight than smoking. On my wish list? That the dangers of thyroid problems and the resulting lifelong battle with hypothyroidism and weight—on top of all the other dangers of smoking— were openly discussed with teenagers before they even start smoking.

Drugs

There are certain drugs that are known to have an effect on thyroid function. These include lithium and the heart drug amiodarone (Cordarone™). If you are taking these drugs now, or have taken them in the past, you are at increased risk for hypothyroidism.

Supplements and Iodine

Certain supplements also increase the risk of thyroid disease. If you are taking too much iodine or iodine-containing herbs such as kelp, bladderwrack, or bugleweed, then you may be creating an increased risk for hypothyroidism. Note, too, that many multivitamins, glandular support formulas, and combination products contain these supplements as well.

Overconsumption of Goitrogenic Foods

There is a certain class of foods called goitrogens that, when eaten in large quantities, can promote goiters and resulting hypothyroidism. Goitrogens are a concern only for people who still have a thyroid and are considered a problem when served raw. It's believed that thorough cooking may minimize or eliminate goitrogenic potential. Goitrogenic foods include brussels sprouts, rutabaga, turnips, kohlrabi, radishes, cauliflower, African cassava, millet, babassu (a palm-tree coconut fruit popular in Brazil and Africa), cabbage, kale, and soy products.

Overconsumption of Soy Products

Soy products, which have become increasingly popular due to a number of reported health benefits, are also being found to have a definite antithyroid and goitrogenic effect. Research is beginning to show that long-term consumption of soy products can promote formation of goiters and development of autoimmune thyroid disease. This is of particular concern for infants on a diet solely consisting of soy-based formula, but is also an issue for adults who regularly eat soy products in various forms, who take soy or isoflavone supplements, or who regularly use soy protein powders. I discuss this in depth in the Epilogue.

Environmental Exposures

Some experts feel that fluoride, such as that found in drinking water and toothpaste, and chlorine in drinking water can interfere with proper thyroid hormone conversion, and result in hypothyroidism. Their recommendation is to drink only distilled water to avoid this problem. This is a controversial recommendation, given that most health practioners feel that children in particular need fluoride in order to avoid the risk of tooth decay and tooth loss. There is also a concern on the part of some alternative practitioners that mecury, a component in dental fillings, can disable the thyroid's ability to convert T4 to T3, resulting in hypothyroidism.

Radiation or Nasal Radium Treatments

During the period from the 1920s through the middle of the 1960s, x-ray treatments to the head, neck, and chest were used as a treatment for tonsils, adenoids, lymph nodes, and thymus gland problems, as well as acne. There is a relationship between these treatments and irregularities in the thyroid gland, including hypothyroidism. X-ray treatment in childhood for malignant conditions such as Hodgkin's disease and throat cancer may also be linked to later development of thyroid nodules and hypothyroidism. Use of these treatments was discontinued for the most part in the mid-1960s. (Do not confuse these treatments with ultraviolet treatments for acne or regular diagnostic x-rays, such as dental x-rays.)

Also, during the 1940s through 1960s, there was a treatment used for tonsillitis, colds, recurrent adenoid problems, and for military submariners and pilots who had trouble with changes in pressure. This treatment, nasal radium therapy, inserted a rod containing 50 milligrams of radium in the nose. The rod was pushed through each nostril and placed against the opening of the eustachian tubes for six to twelve minutes. Repeated over a period of months, this would shrink tissues. An estimated 67,000 Marylanders received nasal radium therapy, and thousands of submariners, pilots, and children of military personnel got the treatments. In recent years, there have been apparent links between radium treatments and thyroid and other immune disorders and health problems.

Severe Snakebite

Not too many people will face life-threatening illness due to snakebite, but it's known that severe illness due to snakebite can result in pituitary damage that causes hypothyroidism. This is reported in people who suffered nearly fatal bites from some rare and highly poisonous vipers and rattlesnakes.

Neck Trauma/Whiplash

Some research has suggested that trauma to the neck, such as whiplash from a car accident or a broken neck, can result in hypothyroidism. Researchers speculate that this may be due to injury to the thyroid tissues themselves.

Nuclear Plant Exposure

Nuclear plants can accidentally release radioactive materials that are damaging to the thyroid. If you lived in or were visiting the area near the Chernobyl plant in the period after the nuclear accident—April 26, 1986—then you are at an increased risk for thyroid problems. The main countries at risk included Belarus, Russian

Federation, and Ukraine. There is a risk, though reduced, to Poland, Austria, Denmark, Finland, Germany, Greece, and Italy.

You may have also been exposed to potentially thyroid-
damaging radioactive materials if you lived near or in the area
downwind from the former nuclear weapons plant at Hanford in
south central Washington state during the 1940s through 1960s,
particularly 1955 to 1965. Hanford released radioactive materials,
including iodine-131, which concentrates in the thyroid gland and
can cause thyroid disease.

During the 1950s and 1960s, approximately 100 nuclear bomb
tests were conducted at the Nevada Nuclear Test Site northwest
of Las Vegas. The fallout from the tests was most concentrated in
counties of western states located east and north of the test site,
such as Utah, Idaho, Montana, Colorado, and Missouri. Exposure
to this fallout increases the risk of thyroid cancer, particularly in
the Farm Belt where children drank fallout-contaminated milk.
There are also cases of autoimmune thyroid problems in the U.S.
that may be due to the iodine-131 released during these nuclear
tests.

Connie's mother lived less than 100 miles from the Nevada
test site:

> As a kid, my mother used to sit outside and watch the nuclear cloud
> float over her school. We even have home movies of her running after
> the "cloud." Not surprisingly, my mom now has thyroid problems I
> believe are directly linked to her exposure.

Several years ago, the newspaper *The Tennessean* presented the
results of an effort to investigate a mysterious pattern of illnesses
that seem to have been concentrated around the Oak Ridge nuclear
facility in Eastern Tennessee. This same pattern was, according to
the newspaper, repeated at other nuclear facilities in Tennessee,
Colorado, South Carolina, New Mexico, Idaho, New York, California,
Ohio, Kentucky, Texas, and Washington state. A number of the people interviewed for *The Tennessean*'s story reported thyroid-related
illnesses they believe are a result of proximity to these nuclear facilities, and possible low-level iodine-131 exposure.

Perchlorate Exposure

Perchlorate is a chemical that blocks iodine from entering the thyroid, and prevents further synthesis of thyroid hormone. There is some evidence and concern that long-term exposure to concentrations of perchlorate—which are found in various water supplies around the nation, particularly in areas near rocket fuel or fireworks plants—can eventually interfere with proper thyroid function and cause increased rates of congenital hypothyroidism in newborns.

Larry L. Ladd, a water quality activist who lives next to America's largest rocket factory, is a key advocate for public awareness on the issue of perchlorate and its potential danger to the thyroid:

> It's well established that fairly low doses of perchlorate can affect a rat's thyroid gland. The same concentrations of perchlorate are now being found in our food and water supply. Are these long-term, low-level exposures harmful to fetuses, growing children, and people with pre-existing thyroid conditions? You cannot be certain until all of the issues of perchlorate toxicology are thoroughly researched, and the scientific studies will not be done unless a concerned public asks for answers.

Exposure to Other Toxic Chemicals

Understanding how long-term exposure to toxic chemicals affects the thyroid is really just beginning. Scientists are beginning to study the effect of certain chemicals on our endocrine glands and the thyroid in particular. But there's strong evidence that exposure to certain toxic chemicals may increase the risk of developing thyroid disease. Some of the chemicals of concern include dioxins, Methyl Tertiary Butyl—known as MTBE—an oxygenate added to gasoline, and other chemicals that act as "endocrine disruptors." A long list of chemicals known to be disruptive or toxic to the immune system and/or thyroid-toxic is available at the Chemical Scorecard Web site, http://www.scorecard.org.

ILLNESSES THAT CAN RAISE THE SUSPICION OF HYPOTHYROIDISM

A number of conditions are known to be more common in people with hypothyroidism, and/or are more difficult to treat and/or resistant to standard medications. When you have one of these problems, and particularly if it is not responding to treatment, you have a greater possibility of being hypothyroid and should have your thyroid evaluated to rule out an underlying disorder.

Carpal Tunnel Syndrome and Tendinitis

If you have carpal tunnel syndrome (CTS), there's a chance that it may be caused by hypothyroidism. CTS is what is known as a repetitive strain injury (RSI). In CTS, the carpal tunnel—a tunnel of bones and ligaments in the wrist—pinches nerves that go to the fingers and thumb, with inflammation of tendons in the wrist. CTS can cause burning, tingling, pain, achiness or numbness in the wrist, fingers or forearm, as well as burning especially in the thumb, index, and middle fingers. CTS can also make it difficult to grip, make a fist, or even hold a cup. A study in 1998 showed that many people with CTS might have unrecognized medical diseases, including hypothyroidism, as the cause of their CTS. If you have CTS, or any form of tendinitis, but have not been diagnosed with or tested for thyroid disease, these new findings suggest that your doctor should order a thyroid function test—among other tests for other diseases implicated in CTS, such as diabetes mellitus, and various arthritis conditions—before starting on other treatments for your CTS.

Polycystic Ovary Syndrome (PCOS)

Polycystic ovary syndrome (PCOS) is a common disease that affects about five percent of younger women. The syndrome is diagnosed when there are longstanding symptoms, such as ovulation problems, infertility, heavy/irregular/absent periods, high levels of male-type hormones (androgens), and small cysts around the ovaries. PCOS is also associated with insulin resistance and is more common in overweight women. Autoimmune thyroid disease and hypothyroidism are more common in women who have PCOS.

Mitral Valve Prolapse (MVP)

If you have been diagnosed with mitral valve prolapse (MVP), you have a greater chance of also having autoimmune thyroid disorders such as Graves' disease and Hashimoto's thyroiditis. MVP is also sometimes known as click-murmur syndrome, Barlow's syndrome, balloon mitral valve, or floppy-valve syndrome. MVP is the most common heart valve abnormality. Some estimates point to two million or more Americans with MVP and most are women (about 80 percent). When you have MVP, one or both flaps of the mitral valve—one of the heart's four valves—are enlarged. Then, when the heart contracts or pumps, the flaps don't close properly, and small amounts of blood can leak backward through the valve and may cause a heart murmur. Typical symptoms of MVP are a pounding sensation, fast heartbeat, palpitations, fatigue, weakness, low tolerance for exercise, chest pain, panic attacks, headaches, migraines, sleeplessness, dizziness, fainting, intestinal problems, and shortness of breath.

I've always had fluttering heartbeat feelings, palpitations (especially after caffeine), shortness of breath, and other MVP symptoms, but my regular doctor had never heard anything unusual in my heart. My MVP was discovered by an internist during a physical. He prides himself on picking up hard-to-define murmurs. He listened to my heart for a few moments and detected the characteristic "click" of a prolapsing mitral valve. A trip to the cardiologist for an echocardiogram confirmed the murmur. The main thing I was told to do? Take antibiotics per his instruction before and after dental work and let any doctors know that I had MVP before surgeries so they can administer antibiotics. I also received a prescription for Atenolol, a beta-blocker. The cardiologist said I should take it if I was having palpitations that were noticeable or prolonged. I rarely have had to use it since the diagnosis, but I do try to minimize my caffeine intake, as this seems to aggravate my MVP.

Depression

Depression is discussed in great depth in upcoming chapters, but it's important to note that ongoing depression, and particularly depression that is resistant to antidepressant treatments, can frequently be a symptom of hypothyroidism.

Other Factors?

There is no question that as researchers begin to understand more about the cause of autoimmune diseases, we'll find out more about how some thyroid diseases develop and why they seem to have become more prevalent in recent years. Deficiencies in certain vitamins, enzymes, or minerals, or overconsumption and overexposure to certain foods and chemicals, may be discovered to play integral roles in thyroid function and health. It's certain, however, that more chemicals in our water or our environment will definitely be linked to the rise in autoimmunity and thyroid dysfunction.

CHAPTER 3

What Are the Symptoms and Signs of Hypothyroidism?

As long as one keeps searching, the answers come.
JOAN BAEZ

If you compare brochures and articles about hypothyroidism, you'll find there is a standard list of "typical" hypothyroid symptoms. For example, the Thyroid Foundation of America lists:

> [feeling] run down, slow, depressed, sluggish, cold, tired . . . lose interest in normal daily activities . . . dryness and brittleness of hair, dry and itchy skin, constipation, muscle cramps, and increased menstrual flow in women.

While these symptoms should raise the suspicion of hypothyroidism in any well-trained doctor, it's also safe to say that this list is just the tiniest tip of a very deep and very large iceberg.

Joyce touches upon some of the many symptoms people experience with hypothyroidism:

> The most irritating thing about hypothyroidism is its fickle and lackadaisical onset. Go figure, a few extra pounds here, a feeling of sluggishness there, so what? Toss in what I affectionately coin, "Brillo hair and prune skin," and the red flags start to push through the cerebral cortex. Gradually, a few other little annoyances stealthily creep in, more bothersome than anything. When you look in the mirror in the morning you wonder, who in the hell stole the outer half of my eyebrows? What in the holy heck happened to my cheek-

bones? My face is so bloated, I look like a beached whale! Or your significant other asks casually, "Why do you have on two pairs of socks, an extra sweatshirt, and your bathrobe when it is 70 degrees in here?"

The symptoms of hypothyroidism can frequently become more severe as the TSH level rises. The number and severity of symptoms, however, appears to be unique to each individual. Some people suffer terribly at a TSH of 15. Others have written to me about "not feeling quite up to par," only to discover that they have a TSH of over 200.

The short symptoms lists found in the conventional brochures never seem comprehensive enough to capture the many symptoms sufferers experience. Therefore, I conducted a survey of 150 hypothyroid patients, who described the symptoms they experienced when their TSH levels rose above normal range. In addition, I used a variety of respected sources—such as *The Merck Manual, American Family Physician Magazine,* information from the Thyroid Foundation of America, and the American Association of Clinical Endocrinologists, and the *Journal of Clinical Endocrinology and Metabolism*—to help develop this list.

HYPOTHYROIDISM SYMPTOMS

Weight Gain (or Sometimes Loss)

Gaining weight inappropriately, or the inability to lose weight, are key symptoms of hypothyroidism. In my case, despite a low-fat, low-calorie diet, and an hour of stationary cycling each night, I was still gaining a pound or two a week during my most hypothyroid state. This is what I call inappropriate weight gain. Later, while still hypothyroid in the high normal TSH range for my lab (TSH of 5 to 6), I went on Weight Watchers™. I followed the program to the letter and usually gained a half-pound or pound a week, while others lost two to three pounds each week.

If you find yourself suddenly gaining weight, or unable to lose weight following a reasonable diet—of course I don't mean cutting

out dessert once a week and expecting to drop pounds and inches—
then this may be a symptom of hypothyroidism.

Don't always expect doctors to believe you, however. Kathryn
had a long and difficult struggle with weight gain before her diagnosis of hypothyroidism:

> When I mentioned the possibility of thyroid disease to a former doc,
> and that my maternal grandmother and mother both are and were
> hypothyroid, he laughed it off and told me to lay off the chips and
> cookies! I was barely eating at that time because I was too tired to
> make it to the kitchen after work.

While weight gain is more common, and weight loss is more
often associated with the overactive metabolism of hyperthyroidism,
you may lose weight when hypothyroid. You could find it hard to
maintain your weight, or lose weight faster than usual, or find yourselves eating more to maintain your weight.

The relationship of hypothyroidism and weight is discussed in
greater depth in chapter 9.

Digestive Problems and Constipation

Constipation is a common symptom of hypothyroidism. Often, this
type of constipation does not respond to increased dietary fiber,
increased water consumption, laxatives, and fiber products like
Metamucil.

Low Body Temperature, Feeling Cold

Feeling cold is a common symptom of hypothyroidism. You may
feel cold when others are feeling hot, or you may always wear socks
to bed, or need a sweater in the summer. In particular, you may
find that your hands and feet are affected. Hypothermia (low body
temperature) is also listed as a symptom of thyroid disease in many
patient informational sources.

Some doctors use basal body temperature—either in conjunction with, or even in some cases, instead of TSH tests—as a way
to diagnose hypothyroidism. This method was initially promoted by
Dr. Broda Barnes. Basal body temperature is the temperature after

awaking and before rising from bed and before any major movement. According to Dr. Barnes and followers of his theories, a basal
body temperature lower than 97.8 to 98.2 degrees Fahrenheit can
be indicative of hypothyroidism.

Tiredness and Weakness

However you describe it, fatigue, exhaustion, weakness, lethargy,
or feeling run down, sluggish, overtired, or just plain pooped out
is one of the most common symptoms of hypothyroidism. You may
find yourself needing a nap in the afternoon just to make it to
dinnertime. You may sleep ten or twelve hours a night and still
wake up exhausted. You may find yourself less able to exercise, and
your endurance drops because of weakness or lethargy. Or you just
walk around spaced out on the same amount of sleep that used to
leave you feeling refreshed.

Exhaustion is also a symptom of sleep deprivation, so it can often
be overlooked by doctors as a sign of a thyroid problem. Average
Americans get only seven hours of sleep each night; so sleep deprivation is a common problem that doctors are likely to assume is the
main reason for your chronic tiredness, not hypothyroidism.

Michele was never much of a sleeper until her thyroid started
becoming underactive:

> Last year, when I began feeling exhausted mid-afternoon, I thought
> something was off. Initially I actually thought I might be pregnant,
> as that was the only time in my life I remember feeling so drained.
> When it got to the point that I was taking naps in the parking lot, I
> headed to the doctor. Interestingly enough, my mom and sister both
> have thyroid problems. My mom got extremely sick when she was
> close to my age and my sister started at a very young age. I didn't
> have a clue that thyroid problems were hereditary, so they didn't pop
> up on my radar screen.

Brain Fog

Brain fog is that fuzzy feeling that makes it difficult to concentrate,
remember things, or focus your mind. Joyce experienced severe
bouts of brain fog as a symptom of her hypothyroidism:

Before hypothyroidism hit, I made lists in my head—I remembered everything, it was like my mind had a computer in it. As my symptoms progressed, I had lists everywhere. Lists that told me what I had to do because I couldn't remember. Lists for tasks, lists for groceries, lists for appointments, lists to remember where I put the lists. When your thyroid is out of whack, you get something I call "Cotton-ball" brain syndrome. That's how it feels, like your head is packed full of cotton balls and absolutely nothing else.

Slow Pulse and Low Blood Pressure

Pulse, or heart rate, varies depending on age, level of fitness, and other factors. But, generally, an average heart rate/pulse runs around 60 to 85 beats per minute. If you are not taking certain drugs that can lower pulse, or you're not in particularly good physical condition (a well-trained athlete can have a normal pulse of 40 to 60 beats per minute) and your pulse is slower than 60 to 85 beats per minute, it can be a symptom of hypothyroidism.

According to the National Institutes of Health, a blood pressure about 120/80 is considered a normal level for most adults. A level, such as 105/65 mm, for example, is considered somewhat "low." Low blood pressure can, in some cases, be a symptom of hypothyroidism.

High Cholesterol Levels

Having unusually high cholesterol levels can be a symptom of underlying hypothyroidism. Some people have reported that despite normal diets, their cholesterol levels reached 300 to 500 points, but returned to normal or only slightly elevated levels once underlying hypothyroidism was treated. If you have high cholesterol that is not responding to diet or cholesterol-lowering drugs, hypothyroidism may be a factor.

Hair/Skin/Nail Problems

Problems with hair, skin, and nails are frequent symptoms of hypothyroidism. Your hair—including body hair and head hair—may be falling out at the root faster than normal and become more brittle, breaking more easily when handled. Your hair can also look and feel very coarse, rough, and dry. You may also notice that you're losing the hair from the outer part of your eyebrow, which is considered a distinct symptom of hypothyroidism, as well as losing eyelashes.

Skin changes are another symptom of hypothyroidism. Skin can become rough, coarse, dry, scaly, itchy, or thick in patches. Your skin can also break out more easily. Nails can also develop problems as a symptom of hypothyroidism. They can become dry, brittle, and may break more easily than normal.

Low, Husky Voice

Changes in voice can be a symptom of hypothyroidism. Most typically, the voice becomes hoarse, husky, or gravelly. Some women have even reported that when hypothyroid, they are mistaken for a man on the phone.

Muscle and Joint Aches and Pains

Pains, aches, and stiffness in various joints and muscles, particularly the hands and feet, often occurs with hypothyroidism. Your aches and pains can sometimes be so severe that doctors mistake them for arthritis symptoms, or diagnose you as having fibromyalgia.

Menstrual Changes or Fertility Problems

Irregularities in your menstrual cycle are more common when hypothyroid. These can include longer periods than are usual for you, or heavier periods than normal, a shorter cycle, or less regular cycle. For example, before I was hypothyroid, I was very regular every twenty-eight days, with a five-day period. The first two days were heavier, tapering to a very light flow from days three to five.

When I became hypothyroid and before my TSH was in the low normal range, my periods starting coming every twenty-one to twenty-four days, lasting up to seven days, and were extremely heavy for four to five days. Now that I'm back to a low normal TSH, my period comes every twenty-six days, lasts five days, and though heavier than before my thyroid problems, it's not as heavy as when I am more hypothyroid.

Difficulty becoming pregnant can sometimes lead a woman to discover previously undiagnosed hypothyroidism. For some women, hypothyroidism can prevent ovulation all or some of the time. Hypothyroidism can also delay the timing of ovulation, and has also been associated with polycystic ovary syndrome (PCO), which is also associated with infertility problems.

Hypothyroidism can increase your risk of miscarriage, and therefore, miscarriage can be considered in some ways a "symptom" of undiagnosed hypothyroidism as well.

Mood, Depression, Thinking

One of the most common symptoms of hypothyroidism is a change in mood, typically a feeling of depression. You might have periods when you feel down, sad, or even mistakenly be diagnosed as clinically depressed instead of hypothyroid. The mood changes associated with hypothyroidism may make you feel restless, or your moods may change easily. You may have feelings of worthlessness, difficulty concentrating, or feel like your brain or mind is "in a fog." You may lose interest in normal daily activities, or be more forgetful and have a tougher time keeping up with work, or schedules, or details.

Hypothyroidism may also be the reason why your antidepressant doesn't seem to be working. In 1997, there were an estimated twenty-five million people in the United States taking antidepressants. And some studies estimate that 80 percent of people on antidepressants report a variety of unresolved symptoms—such as weight gain, lethargy, and loss of libido—that are also very common symptoms of thyroid disease. A significant percentage of people on antidepressants could actually be suffering from an undiagnosed thyroid problem.

Low Sex Drive

Having what doctors refer to as low libido—and what the rest of us refer to as low sex drive, or no sizzle between the sheets—is a common, but not as often discussed, symptom of hypothyroidism.

This applies equally to men and women, and in fact, is often the symptom that commonly leads men to a diagnosis. Interestingly, major research published in the *Journal of the American Medical Association* in early 1999 found that about 43 percent of women and 31 percent of men suffer "sexual inadequacy" for a variety of reasons, including: low desire, performance anxiety, premature ejaculation, among other concerns. Research indicated that many of these sexual concerns were probably treatable, as they are due to physical and health issues, including hormonal imbalances such as hypothyroidism.

Eye Problems

There is a form of eye disease, called thyroid eye disease, also known as Graves' ophthalmopathy or thyroid associated ophthalmopathy (TAO). Thyroid eye disease is most often associated with Graves' disease. Thyroid eye disease is an inflammation of the eyes, with swelling of the tissues around the eyes, and bulging of the eyes. In the majority of cases, this inflammation will not cause serious or permanent trouble. Early signs include:

- bulging of the eyes due to inflammation of the tissues behind the eyeball (the medical term is exophthalmos)
- blurred or diminished vision
- red or inflamed eyes
- double vision

Many experts believe that the swelling is caused by antibodies attacking the tissues of the eye muscles. There may also be a sensitivity to light and a continual feeling that there is something foreign or gritty in the eyes. Ultimately, the eyeball may protrude because tissues behind the eye swell and become inflamed, pushing the eyeball forward. The front surface of the eye may become dry.

While thyroid eye disease is most associated with Graves' disease, hypothyroidism seems to create a variety of other irritating eye problems. You may experience the following eye symptoms:

- Eyes that feel gritty and dry
- Eyes that are photosensitive or sensitive to light
- Eyes that get jumpy, or have more frequent tics, sometimes referred to as "nystagmus"
- A rapidly shifting gaze makes you feel dizzy or feel vertigo
- Sensitivity of eyes creates headaches
- Eyes that feel gritty or achy
- Eyes that are dry and blurry
- Eyes that are dry and blurry but relieved by drops or liquid tears

Neck and Throat Complaints

A goiter, swelling or thickness in the neck is a fairly obvious sign of a potential thyroid problem. However, even in the absence of a goiter or swelling that a doctor can feel, you may have strange feelings in the neck or throat. These feelings have been described as "fullness," discomfort with neckties or clothing around the neck, a sense of neck or throat pressure, a choking sensation, a feeling like something is stuck in the throat, or difficulty swallowing.

Hearing/Tinnitus

According to researchers, the incidence of tinnitus can be correlated to the severity of hypothyroidism. Tinnitus is a problem that makes it seem as if you are hearing something—in some cases hissing, roaring, whistling, clicking, ringing—when there is no sound. It is most commonly referred to as "ringing in the ears." Tinnitus can be a debilitating problem for some people, and the American Tinnitus Association estimates that over 50 million Americans are affected by tinnitus to some degree, and twelve million suffer severely enough to seek medical attention for the problem.

More Infections and Lowered Resistance

Some doctors believe that more frequent infections, or less resistance to infection, are symptoms of hypothyroidism. Many people with thyroid problems also report getting more frequent colds, flus and sinus infections, and have a longer, harder time recuperating from these infections.

Allergies

Development of allergies, or worsening of existing allergies—including hay fever, seasonal allergies, and food allergies—have all been reported as symptoms of hypothyroidism.

Sleep Apnea and Snoring

Snoring can be a symptom of sleep apnea, and sleep apnea can be a symptom of hypothyroidism. Sleep apnea involves momentary lapses of breathing while sleeping and is accompanied by loud snoring, gasping for breath as you sleep, and feeling tired all the time, no matter how much sleep you get.

Breathing Difficulties and Asthma-Like Feelings

While not reported in patient literature, a hypothyroidism symptom that many people have reported to me—and one I experience myself—is a feeling of shortness of breath and tightness in the chest. Some people describe this feeling as "I feel like I need to yawn hard to even get enough oxygen." Sometimes this can be mistaken for asthma, which is what they initially told me. But my doctor felt it was inaccurate because it wasn't accompanied by any wheezing that is typical of asthma. I also noticed it was only a problem when I was in high normal range or out of range and at hypothyroid TSH levels.

Dizziness and Vertigo

Vertigo is dizziness with the illusion of motion. When you have vertigo, you may feel you are moving, or that things are moving around you. Lightheadedness, dizziness, and vertigo can all be symptoms of hypothyroidism. Typically, these symptoms are usually worse with higher TSH levels.

Puffiness and Swelling

Swelling and puffiness—referred to by doctors as "edema"—of various parts of the body can be symptoms of hypothyroidism. In particular, puffiness and swelling may affect the eyes, eyelids, and face, and can sometimes be most painful and visible in feet and hands.

SPECIAL NOTE: INFANT AND CHILDREN'S HYPOTHYROIDISM SYMPTOMS

Symptoms of hypothyroidism in infants include a puffy face, swollen tongue, hoarse cry, cold extremities, mottled skin, low muscle tone, poor feeding, thick coarse hair that grows low on the forehead, a large soft spot, prolonged jaundice, a herniated belly button, lethargy, sleeping most of the time, appearing tired even when awake, persistent constipation, looking bloated or full to the touch, and little to no growth.

In children, symptoms are primarily a lack of growth, but can also include school problems, a diagnosis of attention deficit disorder, delayed puberty, and many of the other symptoms that adults experience, including unusual fatigue, weight gain, constipation, sensitivity to cold, dry skin, and hair loss.

❀   ❀   ❀

While this list of symptoms typically exceeds most of the standard symptom lists you'll find in patient educational materials, it is *still* by no means inclusive. You may have unique symptoms that are specific to your own hypothyroidism and health. One way to get to know your own symptoms better is by keeping a journal or charting your symptoms according to time of day, time of the month, and other variables such as exercise, diet, supplements, and any blood test values you have. This can help you better understand your body's unique response to hypothyroidism.

CHAPTER 4

Hypothyroidism Diagnosis and Symptoms Checklist

Nothing in life is to be feared. It is only to be understood.
MARIE CURIE

The following checklist can help you communicate your risk factors and symptoms to your doctor, as an aid in getting a proper diagnosis of hypothyroidism. It can also serve as background information in your discussions regarding finetuning your dosage. You need to be at the optimal TSH level for your own wellness. At the end of this chapter, I've also included basal body and Wilson's Syndrome temperature charts that you can use to track your own temperatures and show to your doctor. I suggest you make a copy of this chapter for yourself to fill out and show to your doctor, and be sure to bring an extra copy for your doctor's files.

✔ I HAVE THE FOLLOWING RISK FACTORS FOR HYPOTHYROIDISM:

Thyroid-Related
❑ My family (parent, sibling, child) has a history of thyroid disease.
❑ My thyroid has been "monitored" in the past due to irregularities.
❑ I've been treated in the past for thyroid disease.
❑ I've been previously diagnosed with and/or treated for goiters/nodules.
❑ In the past, I tested positive for thyroid antibodies.
❑ In the past, I've been treated for hypothyroidism.

❑ A doctor has prescribed thyroid hormone for me in the past.

❑ I had thyroid problems during or after a pregnancy.

❑ In the past, I have had a problem with my thyroid that resolved itself without further treatment. (I have had a diagnosis of a "temporary, or transient, thyroiditis" or "transient hypothyroidism".)

❑ I currently have a goiter or nodules.

❑ I have had part/all of my thyroid removed (a thyroidectomy) due to cancer.

❑ I have had part/all of my thyroid removed due to nodules or goiter.

❑ I have had part/all of my thyroid removed as a treatment for Graves' disease/hyperthyroidism.

❑ I have been treated with radioactive iodine (RAI) for Graves' disease/hyperthyroidism or thyroid cancer.

❑ I was treated with antithyroid drugs (i.e., Tapazole or PTU) due to Graves' disease/hyperthyroidism.

Endocrine-Related

❑ I have or had a pituitary tumor and/or pituitary disease.

Autoimmune Diseases

❑ I have chronic fatigue syndrome (CFS) and/or fibromyalgia.

❑ Member(s) of my family (parent, sibling, child) have CFS and/or fibromyalgia.

❑ I have another autoimmune disease (i.e, Crohn's disease, insulin-dependent (type I) diabetes, multiple sclerosis, pernicious anemia, scleroderma, Sjögren's syndrome, lupus, and others).

❑ Member(s) of my family (parent, sibling, child) has/had another autoimmune disease.

Age

❑ I am over 60.

Female-Specific

❑ I am female.

❑ I am perimenopausal or menopausal.

❑ I have had a baby in the past nine months.

❑ I have a history of more than one miscarriage.

❑ I have a history of infertility.

Smoking

❑ I am currently a smoker.
❑ I've recently quit smoking.
❑ I was a smoker in the past.

Drugs and Supplements

❑ I have been treated with lithium, amiodarone (Cordarone), or iodine in the past or am currently being treated with these drugs.
❑ I have been self-treating with iodine, kelp, bladderwrack, and/or bugleweed.

Radiation or Radium Treatments

❑ I have had radiation treatment to my head, neck, or chest.
❑ I have had radiation treatment to treat my tonsils, adenoids, lymph nodes, thymus gland problems, or acne.
❑ I have had numerous x-ray treatments (not dental or diagnostic x-rays) to the head and neck.
❑ I had "Nasal Radium Therapy" sometime during the 1940s through 1960s, as a treatment for tonsillitis, colds, and other ailments or as a military submariner and/or pilot who had trouble with drastic changes in pressure.

Diet

❑ I consume substantial quantities of any of the following foods: brussels sprouts, rutabaga, turnips, kohlrabi, radishes, cauliflower, African cassava, millet, babassu (a palm-tree coconut fruit popular in Brazil and Africa) cabbage, and kale.
❑ I eat substantial quantities of soy products, i.e., tofu, soy milk, soy protein, soy capsules, and soy powders.

Snakebite

❑ I have had a severe or life-threatening snakebite in the past.

Neck Trauma

❑ I have had serious trauma to the neck, such as whiplash from a car accident.

Chemical Exposure
❑ I live near a plant that produces rocket fuel, or my work exposes me to the chemical perchlorate.

Nuclear Exposure
❑ I lived, or live, near a nuclear plant.
❑ I lived, or was visiting, in or around Chernobyl in the weeks after the nuclear accident, which occurred on April 26, 1986. (Main countries at risk included Belarus, Russian Federation, Ukraine. Lesser risk to Poland, Austria, Denmark, Finland, Germany, Greece, Italy.)
❑ I lived in, near, or downwind from the former nuclear weapons plant at Hanford in south central Washington state in the 1940s through 1960s, but particularly during the period 1955 to 1965.
❑ I lived near or in the general region of the Nevada Nuclear Test Site in the 1950s and 1960s. According to the National Cancer Institute, the highest per capita thyroid doses of radiation were obtained in counties of western states located east and north of the NTS, such as Utah, Idaho, Montana, Colorado, and Missouri.

I currently have, or have in the past, been diagnosed with the following diseases or conditions, known to occur more frequently in people with thyroid disease
❑ carpal tunnel syndrome/tendonitis
❑ polycystic ovary syndrome (PCOS)
❑ mitral valve prolapse (MVP) (heart murmur, palpitations)
❑ Epstein-Barr virus (EBV)
❑ mononucleosis
❑ depression

✔ I HAVE THE FOLLOWING SYMPTOMS OF HYPOTHYROIDISM

Weight Gain (or Loss)
❑ I am gaining weight inappropriately.
❑ I'm unable to lose weight with proper diet/exercise.
❑ I'm losing weight inappropriately.

Digestive Problems/Constipation
❏ I am constipated, sometimes severely.

Body Temperature
❏ I have been diagnosed as having hypothermia (low body temperature).
❏ My "normal" basal body temperature is lower than 97.8 to 98.2 degrees Fahrenheit.
❏ I feel cold when others feel hot. I need extra sweaters when others need air conditioning.
❏ I feel cold, especially in the hands and/or feet.

Tiredness/Weakness
❏ I feel fatigued more than normal.
❏ I feel weak.
❏ I feel run down, sluggish, lethargic.
❏ I feel like I can't get enough sleep, even though I'm sleeping the amount I honestly need to feel well-rested.

Pulse/Blood Pressure
❏ I have a slow pulse.
❏ I have low blood pressure.

Cholesterol Levels
❏ I have high cholesterol.
❏ I have high cholesterol that is resistant to diet or drug treatment.

Hair/Skin/Nails
❏ My hair is rough, coarse, dry, breaking, brittle.
❏ My hair is falling out more than usual.
❏ My eyebrows or eyelashes are falling out.
❏ My skin is rough, coarse, dry, scaly, itchy, and thick.
❏ My nails have been dry, brittle, and break more easily.
❏ My skin is breaking out.

Voice
❏ My voice has become hoarse, husky, or gravelly.

Aches and Pains
❏ I have pains, aches, and stiffness in various joints, hands, and feet.
❏ I have developed carpal-tunnel syndrome, or my existing carpal tunnel syndrome is getting worse.

Fertility/Menstruation
❏ I am having irregular menstrual cycles (longer, or heavier, or more frequent).
❏ I am having trouble conceiving a baby.
❏ I have started to develop ovarian cysts.
❏ I have a history of one or more miscarriages.

Mood/Depression/Thinking
❏ I feel depressed.
❏ I feel restless.
❏ My moods change easily.
❏ I have feelings of worthlessness.
❏ I have difficulty concentrating.
❏ I have feelings of sadness.
❏ I'm taking an antidepressant, but it doesn't seem to be working.
❏ I seem to be losing interest in normal daily activities.
❏ I'm more forgetful lately.
❏ My mind feels like I'm in a "fog."

Sex Drive
❏ I have no sex drive or a reduced sex drive.
❏ I have difficulty reaching orgasm.

Eyes
❏ My eyes feel gritty and dry.
❏ My eyes feel sensitive to light.
❏ My eyes get jumpy (tics in eyes), which makes me dizzy (vertigo) and gives me headaches.

Neck/Throat
❏ I have strange feelings in my neck or throat, for example, a feeling of "fullness," or pressure, a choking sensation, or difficulty swallowing.

❑ I have a lump, or what appears to be some sort of fullness or growth in my neck area.

Hearing/Tinnitus
❑ I have tinnitus (ringing in ears).

Infections/Resistance
❑ I am getting more frequent infections or infections that last longer.
❑ I get recurrent sinus infections.

Allergies
❑ I have developed allergies or my allergies have become worse.

Sleeping/Snoring
❑ I'm snoring more lately.
❑ I have (may have) sleep apnea.

Breathing
❑ I feel shortness of breath and tightness in the chest.
❑ I feel the need to yawn to get oxygen.

Dizziness
❑ I have vertigo.
❑ I feel lightheaded at times.

Puffiness/Swelling
❑ I have puffiness and swelling around the eyes and face.
❑ I have swollen feet.
❑ I have swollen hands.
❑ I have swollen eyelids.

Special Risk/Symptoms List for Infants
❑ My infant is on soy formula.
❑ My infant has family members (parents, siblings) with thyroid disease.
❑ My infant has a puffy face.
❑ My infant has a swollen tongue.
❑ My infant has a hoarse cry.

❑ My infant has cold extremities.
❑ My infant has mottled skin.
❑ My infant has low muscle tone.
❑ My infant is not eating well.
❑ My infant has thick coarse hair that grows low on the forehead.
❑ My infant has a large soft spot.
❑ My infant has had prolonged jaundice.
❑ My infant has a herniated belly button.
❑ My infant is lethargic.
❑ My infant sleeps most of the time.
❑ My infant appears tired even when awake.
❑ My infant has persistent constipation.
❑ My infant is bloated or full to the touch.
❑ My infant has had little to no growth.

Special Symptoms List for Children

❑ My child took soy formula as an infant.
❑ My child has family members (parents, siblings) with thyroid disease.
❑ My child is not keeping up with growth charts for height.
❑ My child is having school problems.
❑ My child has been diagnosed with attention deficit disorder.
❑ My child is having delayed puberty.
❑ My child is unusually fatigued, exhausted, or sleeping far more than usual.
❑ My child is gaining weight inappropriately.
❑ My child is severely constipated.
❑ My child is sensitive to cold.
❑ My child's hair is rough, coarse dry, breaking, brittle.
❑ My child's hair is falling out more than usual.
❑ My child's eyebrows or eyelashes are falling out.
❑ My child's skin is rough, coarse, dry, scaly, itchy, and thick.
❑ My child's voice has become hoarse, husky, or gravelly.
❑ My child is complaining of pains, aches, and stiffness in various joints, hands, and feet.
❑ My child seems depressed.
❑ My child seems restless.
❑ My child has difficulty concentrating.

❑ My child seems to be losing interest in normal daily activities.
❑ My child seems more forgetful lately.
❑ My child complains of strange feelings in the neck or throat, or difficulty swallowing.
❑ My child seems to have some sort of fullness or growth in the neck area.
❑ My child gets more frequent infections or infections that last longer.
❑ My child is snoring more lately.
❑ My child yawns frequently to get oxygen.
❑ My child has puffiness and swelling around the eyes and face.
❑ My child has swollen feet, hands, or eyelids.

✎ BASAL BODY TEMPERATURE CHART

INSTRUCTIONS: Use an oral glass/Mercury thermometer. Shake the thermometer down before going to bed and leave it close by and within reach. As soon as you wake up, with a minimum of movement, put the thermometer in your armpit, next to the skin, and leave it in place for ten minutes. Record the readings for three to five consecutive days. Women who still have their menstrual period should not test on days 1, 2, 3, or 4 of their period, but can begin on day 5. Men, and girls and women who are not menstruating can test any time of the month.

Day 1:_____degrees Fahrenheit (Day of menstrual cycle:_____)

Day 2:_____degrees Fahrenheit (Day of menstrual cycle:_____)

Day 3:_____degrees Fahrenheit (Day of menstrual cycle:_____)

Day 4:_____degrees Fahrenheit (Day of menstrual cycle:_____)

Day 5:_____degrees Fahrenheit (Day of menstrual cycle:_____)

Average temperature: _____ degrees Fahrenheit

✎ WILSON'S SYNDROME TEMPERATURE CHART

INSTRUCTIONS: Use an oral glass/Mercury thermometer. Take your temperature three hours after waking, and then again three hours later, and finally, three hours later.

Day 1: (Day of menstrual cycle: _____)

Time Awoke:_____a.m./p.m.

1st temperature/Time:_____a.m./p.m._____degrees Fahrenheit

2nd temperature/Time:_____a.m./p.m._____degrees Fahrenheit

3rd temperature/Time:_____a.m./p.m._____degrees Fahrenheit

Day 1 Average: _____ degrees Fahrenheit

Day 2: (Day of menstrual cycle: _____)

Time Awoke:_____a.m./p.m.

1st temperature/Time:_____a.m./p.m._____degrees Fahrenheit

2nd temperature/Time:_____a.m./p.m._____degrees Fahrenheit

3rd temperature/Time:_____a.m./p.m._____degrees Fahrenheit

Day 2 Average: _____ degrees Fahrenheit

Day 3: (Day of menstrual cycle: _____)

Time Awoke:_____a.m./p.m.

1st temperature/Time:_____a.m./p.m._____degrees Fahrenheit

2nd temperature/Time:_____a.m./p.m._____degrees Fahrenheit

3rd temperature/Time:_____a.m./p.m._____degrees Fahrenheit

Day 3 Average: _____ degrees Fahrenheit

Day 4: (Day of menstrual cycle: _____)

Time Awoke:_____a.m./p.m.

1st temperature/Time:_____a.m./p.m._____degrees Fahrenheit

2nd temperature/Time:_____a.m./p.m._____degrees Fahrenheit

3rd temperature/Time:_____a.m./p.m._____degrees Fahrenheit

Day 4 Average: _____ degrees Fahrenheit

Day 5: (Day of menstrual cycle: _____)

Time Awoke:_____a.m./p.m.

1st temperature/Time:_____a.m./p.m._____degrees Fahrenheit

2nd temperature/Time:_____a.m./p.m._____degrees Fahrenheit

3rd temperature/Time:_____a.m./p.m._____degrees Fahrenheit

Day 5 Average: _____ degrees Fahrenheit

CHAPTER 5

Hypothyroidism Treatment and Thyroid Hormone Replacement

Medicine is not only a science; it is also an art. It does not consist of compounding pills and plasters; it deals with the very processes of life, which must be understood before they may be guided.
PARACELSUS

Once you have a diagnosis of hypothyroidism, it's useful to sit down with your doctor and make sure that you get answers to some very important questions. Often, this is hard. In the course of an appointment, your doctor might say "Hmm, I'm going to check your thyroid." A nurse draws some blood and next thing you know, you're getting a rushed phone call from the doctor's office, saying that your thyroid's a little low, and they'd like to phone in a prescription for you. Unfortunately, all too often this is how you find out you are hypothyroid, and even more unfortunate, this may be all the information you get from your doctor.

Even if this is how you find out, call back, and ask for a phone call or personal consultation with your doctor to discuss your diagnosis. And don't hang up or leave till you get answers to the following critical questions.

What is the normal TSH range at the lab where you send my blood, and what was my TSH?

In addition to your own TSH level, it is important for you to know the normal TSH values at *your* lab because this number can have a major impact on your ability to live well with hypothyroidism.

What is your idea of an optimum TSH level for me?

This is a basic question, but it is also a loaded question. Your doctor's answer will tell you her or his philosophy about "normal" TSH.

Some doctors believe that getting you into the very top of the normal range is their sole objective, and then the job is done. So, for example, using the 5.5 TSH level from my local lab, that sort of doctor would believe that getting me to 5.4 constitutes full treatment. And if I don't feel well at 5.4, then something else is wrong with me because it's certainly not my thyroid. The majority of conventional doctors seem to follow this philosophy. The idea that different people feel differently at different TSH levels within the range has not gained widespread acceptance among endocrinologists or others treating thyroid disease.

There's also a tendency among some doctors to leave patients in the higher end of the normal range because of their concerns about osteoporosis. There is evidence that untreated hyperthyroidism puts a patient at increased risk of osteoporosis. However, there are also studies that show no greater increased risk of osteoporosis for people on thyroid hormone replacement with TSH in the normal range, and even suppressed to hyperthyroid levels for people who have had thyroid cancer. There is no definitive proof that low or suppressed TSH levels pose a clear risk of osteoporosis, and don't let your doctor tell you that there is.

What thyroid hormone replacement have you prescribed for me?

Since you probably can't read the writing, you'll need to ask! The issue here is, brand name or generic, and if a brand name, did your doctor specify "no generic substitutions." Brand name thyroid hormone replacement is considered more reliable. Generics can be erratic, and should be avoided.

How quickly can we expect my TSH to return to normal, given the dosage you've prescribed?

What you want to know is if your doctor is giving you a small dose of thyroid replacement, and intending to see what happens very slowly, or is he or she going to get you into the normal range as fast as possible. There are reasons for taking both approaches, but it's important to know. Some doctors will put you on a tiny dose, then tell you you'll feel better in two weeks. When two weeks come and go, and you don't feel better, you think something's wrong with *you.*

How often will you test my TSH until I get back to feeling well?

What you want to hear is that the doc is going to stay on top of getting you into normal range. This means probably seeing you every six to eight weeks for a TSH test, followed up with an adjustment to your dosage, until you're feeling better and TSH results are normal.

After I'm feeling well, how often do you suggest I come back for a TSH test to make sure my dosage requirements haven't changed?

If the doc says once a year or longer, start wondering. Most doctors recommend every six months in the first year or two, and every year—at minimum—thereafter.

If I have questions between appointments, how can I best get in touch with you? Do you return calls yourself or do your nurses? Can I fax in a question? Do you have an email address for patient correspondence?

Here, you can gauge how available the doctor plans to be. And if you have the option of looking for another doctor, the response here may help you decide if you'll stay or go. Some doctors will return calls themselves or even answer email. Others will refer all questions to the nurses (who, by the way, often have just as good or even better information. So don't write that off as an option in some cases.) But if you want personalized, hands-on service, listen to what your doctor says here because you'll get an idea of what to expect.

ABOUT THYROID HORMONE TREATMENTS

When you are hypothyroid, your body doesn't produce enough thyroid hormone, and you need to replace that missing thyroid hormone. This process of treating hypothyroidism by taking external thyroid hormone drugs is called "thyroid hormone replacement."

When it comes to thyroid hormone replacement, there are several types of thyroid drugs.

• *Levothyroxine,* which is pronounced lee-voe-thy-ROX-een. This is the generic name for synthetic thyroxine, also known as T4. Brand names in the U.S. and Canada include Synthroid, Levothroid, Levoxyl, Eltroxin, and PMS-Levothyroxine.

• *Liothyronine,* pronounced lye-oh-THY-roe-neen, the synthetic form of triiodothyronine, T3. The brand name in the U.S. and Canada is Cytomel.

• *Liotrix,* pronounced LYE-oh-trix, is a synthetic combination of levothyroxine and liothyronine. It's a synthetic T4/T3 drug. The brand name in the U.S. is Thyrolar.

• *Natural thyroid.* This is nonsynthetic thyroid hormone replacement produced using the thyroid gland of pigs, containing T4, T3, and other nonspecific components of thyroid hormone. The brand names in the U.S. are Armour Thyroid, Naturethroid, and Westhroid.

Levothyroxine/Synthetic T4

The vast majority of doctors prescribe levothyroxine as the thyroid hormone replacement drug of choice, and when they prescribe levothyroxine, it's usually the brand name Synthroid. Synthroid is the top-selling thyroid hormone replacement in the U.S., and one of the top-selling drugs in America. It has a firm hold on the top position due to the manufacturer's extensive marketing to the medical community.

Though your doctor might tell you otherwise, Synthroid is not more effective than the other brand name thyroid hormones, even though it is usually more expensive at many pharmacies. The major brands have been found to be bioequivalent. The main difference is that each brand of levothyroxine has different fillers and binders.

A small number of patients apparently are allergic to the fillers in one versus another. So if you have unusual reactions, such as hives or rashes, or other allergic responses after taking certain brands, you should talk to your doctor about trying a different brand.

Because all the brand-name levothyroxines are considered bioequivalent, you have the option of taking levothyroxine products that aren't as expensive as Synthroid, as long as you remain with a brand name. While all levothyroxine products have some ups and downs in potency from batch to batch, brand names have fewer variations in potency than generic brands. Most doctors do not recommend or prescribe generic levothyroxine anyway, but pharmacies often will substitute them. Some health maintenance organizations insist on the cheaper generic when a brand name has been prescribed. *Do not accept generic levothyroxine if at all possible,* and always be sure to check your prescription every time you get it filled to make sure the pharmacy hasn't substituted generic for brand name.

Liothyronine/Synthetic T3 and Liotrix, Synthetic T3/T4

Synthetic levothyroxine offers only T4 and depends on the body's ability to effectively convert T4 to the T3 needed at the cellular level. If the conversion works properly in the body, the levothyroxine therapy will usually work, as it does for some people with hypothyroidism who do take the pill, feel fine and normal, and only think about their hypothyroidism when they remember to have their blood checked each year.

If there's evidence—in the form of unrelieved symptoms despite normal TSH levels—that the conversion is not optimal, some doctors will prescribe additional T3, typically as Cytomel or time-released, compounded liothyronine, or via the synthetic T4/T3 drug Thyrolar, or natural T4/T3 drugs like Armour.

Doctors who are willing to work with these drugs tend to be osteopaths, naturopaths, and holistic M.D.s. There are some endocrinologists who are using these drugs when necessary for a particular patient's treatment. Psychopharmacologists are also known to use T3 as a way to help treat unrelieved depression in hypothyroid patients and in nonhypothyroid people with resistant depression.

Natural Thyroid

Natural thyroid—which is known by the brands Armour Thyroid, as well as Westhroid and Naturethroid in the U.S.—are natural thyroid products produced from the desiccated thyroid glands of pigs. They contain T4, T3, T1, and T2, as well as other thyroid hormone components. In addition to being in favor with some holistic and natural practitioners, natural thyroid product fans also include some "old-timers," doctors who used natural thyroid successfully for years with their patients, and then saw the health of their patients erode when their patients switched over to synthetics. Naturethroid is a particular brand of natural thyroid hormone that is hypoallergenic and does not include any corn binders.

Taking Your Thyroid Hormone

When you pick up your prescription for thyroid hormone, some pharmacies will send you home with a basic page of information or maybe the drug information insert. Others provide no additional information beyond the label on the pill bottle. Even if you've been taking your thyroid hormone for years or have attempted to read a pharmaceutical company product insert, you should know how to store and take your thyroid hormone and whether there are interactions with foods and other drugs.

What if You Miss a Dose?

All the package instructions say that if you miss a dose, you should take it as soon as possible. If you're close to the time for the next dose, skip the missed dose and just go back to your regular dosing schedule. Basically, you shouldn't double up if you miss a day.

If I miss a dose, I usually split the dose and make it up over the next two days. But that's just me, and that's not medical advice. Ask your doctor what she or he thinks you should do if you miss a dose.

Should You Refrigerate Your Thyroid Hormone?

At present, the only brand of thyroid hormone replacement in pill form that requires refrigeration is Thyrolar, the brand name for liotrix, the synthetic T4/T3 product. This was a new requirement just started in the past several years, though the drug has been on the market far longer. The manufacturer had its last round of evaluations and potency studies on product that was refrigerated, so the law now requires that it list that the product requires refrigeration. Pharmacists at Forest, the manufacturer, have indicated that refrigeration will actually help the product maintain optimal potency longer. If you need to travel, however, they say the product should remain stable for at least a week. So you don't have to go to extraordinary lengths to keep Thyrolar refrigerated while traveling.

The other products have no refrigeration requirement, but, anecdotally, some patients who have taken thyroid hormone for years have told me that they regularly keep it in the refrigerator because they feel that it keeps their prescriptions from losing their potency. Since Thyrolar is synthetic like the other products, if the pharmacists say that refrigerating Thyrolar keeps *it* potent longer, I wonder why that wouldn't be true for the similar products that don't require refrigeration? There are no official proclamations on this from the drug companies, but I can tell you, I refrigerate my Thyrolar, and when I was on levothyroxine products in the past, I refrigerated them too.

Pregnancy and Breastfeeding

Should You Take Thyroid Hormone Replacement When You're Pregnant?

We take seriously the warnings not to take most drugs during pregnancy, and, for the most part, this is very good advice. However, when it comes to thyroid hormone, you're replacing something essential that your body is missing. Thyroid hormone is not something optional; it is absolutely *essential* for your body's proper functioning, and when you are pregnant. It is even more essential for a healthy pregnancy, and to avoid detrimental effects on your baby's developing brain. So *do not stop taking thyroid hormone when pregnant*. If you are taking your thyroid hormone in the proper dose, very little crosses over to the baby, and there's no evidence that it causes any harm to the baby whatsoever. It is considered one of the safest things to take during pregnancy, safer than a decongestant for example. Keep in mind, however, that you are likely to require dosage changes while pregnant.

Can You Take Thyroid Hormone While Breastfeeding?

Thyroid hormone is not something optional; it is absolutely *essential* for your body's proper functioning and is also important to your ability to maintain a milk supply. So do not stop taking thyroid hormone when nursing. If you are taking your thyroid hormone in the proper dose, very little to none enters the baby's milk, and there's no evidence that it causes any harm to the baby whatsoever. Dosage requirements do change in the months after pregnancy for many women, however, so be sure to be checked by your doctor.

How to Take Your Thyroid Hormone

Should You Take Your Thyroid Hormone with Food versus on an Empty Stomach?

If you eat while taking certain prescription drugs, the food in your stomach may delay or reduce the drug's absorption. This is true for thyroid hormone. Food can often slow the process of the drug entering the stomach, but it may also affect absorption of the drug you're taking by binding with it. This decreases the body's ability to absorb the medication by changing the rate at which it dissolves or by changing the stomach's acid balance. Some doctors will tell you it doesn't matter, but if you want to get the most "bang for your buck," thyroid hormone-wise, you'll have best absorption if you take your thyroid hormone first thing the morning, on an empty stomach about one hour before eating.

However, if you don't take it this way, then consistency becomes the key to maintaining a stable level in your bloodstream. If you're going to take your thyroid hormone with food, take it every day with food, consistently. If you've changed from taking it on an empty stomach, you should have another TSH test about six to eight weeks later to ensure you're receiving the proper amount of thyroid hormone. While taking the drug with food might inhibit absorption somewhat, the safety check of an additional blood test will ensure your dosage gets changed as needed. But, again, *consis-*

tency is the key. Don't take it some days with food, some days without, or you're sure to have erratic absorption, and it will be harder to regulate your TSH levels.

What is the Impact of a High-Fiber Diet?

Many people on thyroid replacement therapy are fighting an additional battle to lose weight and switching to a high-fiber diet can be a help in that weight battle. But a high-fiber diet can also affect your thyroid hormone absorption. Anything that affects your digestion speed, or speed of food absorption into the stomach, can affect your absorption of thyroid hormone. Since high-fiber diets are known to speed digestion, they can also inhibit absorption for some people. So, should you forget about eating high-fiber? Absolutely not!

Since the benefits of a high-fiber diet are known, again, the issue is consistency. If you are already eating a high-fiber diet regularly and have regular TSH testing done, your dosage level is appropriate for you, given your diet. If you are starting a new regimen of eating high-fiber, plan to get tested around six to eight weeks after you change your diet, to make sure you're receiving the proper amount of thyroid hormone. But be consistent. Don't jump around or you'll have erratic absorption, and that can wreak havoc on TSH levels . . . *and* how you feel! But, again, you can bypass some of the impact by taking your thyroid hormone first thing in the morning, on an empty stomach, waiting at least an hour to eat. This will ensure maximum absorption *whatever* you're eating!

What About Vitamins with Iron or Iron Supplements?

Iron, whether alone, or as part of a multivitamin or prenatal vitamin supplement, can interfere with thyroid hormone absorption. But don't stop taking your iron. You can still take iron supplements when you're on thyroid hormone replacement. The only concern is that you should *not* take your vitamins with iron at the same time as your thyroid hormone. To ensure there's no interference with absorption, allow *at least two to three hours* between taking iron and thyroid hormone.

What About Calcium Supplements?

Many people on thyroid hormone replacement—especially women concerned about osteoporosis—also take calcium supplements. Calcium supplements are also important for thyroid cancer survivors because the suppressive doses of thyroid hormone called for in cancer patients may increase the risk of osteoporosis. You need to be careful about calcium supplements, however. A 1998 report in the *Journal of the American Medical Association* indicated that the timing of the dosage of thyroid hormone replacement and calcium pills could be a problem.

The report indicated that some patients taking levothyroxine experienced an increase in TSH levels after they started to take calcium supplements. When they changed their pattern and began to take the calcium and thyroid hormone *at least four hours apart*, TSH returned to the initial level. This finding can be of particular relevance to those who have had their thyroid removed and are taking calcium on doctor's orders. The calcium taken at the same time as thyroid hormone was, in some cases, raising TSH above levels recommended to prevent thyroid cancer recurrence.

If you are taking calcium, it should be taken at least *four hours apart* from thyroid hormone.

What About Calcium-Fortified Orange Juice?

Taking thyroid hormone about the same time as calcium-fortified orange juice has reportedly had a similar effect as taking calcium pills with thyroid. If you want to ensure proper dosage and absorption, don't take your thyroid pills at the same time as calcium-fortified orange juice. Keep in mind that you should drink calcium-fortified orange juice and take thyroid hormone at least *four hours apart.*

Is There a Problem with Antacids?

Antacids—like Tums or Mylanta, in liquid or tablet forms—may delay or reduce the absorption of your thyroid hormone. So, again, they should be taken *at least two hours* apart from thyroid hormone.

What About Over-the-Counter Drugs Like Cough Medicines, Cold Medicines, and Decongestants That Recommend "Do Not Take If You Have Thyroid Disease"?

Most packages of over-the-counter cough and cold medicines, and decongestants recommend: "Do not take if you have one of the following . . . " and then go on to list thyroid disease. While you should always check with your doctor, it's generally understood that this warning is intended more for people with an overactive thyroid—hyperthyroidism—than hypothyroidism. Stimulants like pseudoephedrine, the main ingredient in Sudafed and many other cold and allergy medicines, can be dangerous to people with hyperthyroidism, as they can add strain to an already taxed heart.

That said, is there a concern for people with hypothyroidism? There are anecdotal reports of people with thyroid disease becoming extra-sensitive to stimulants. For example, some people with hypothyroidism seem to develop sensitivities to caffeine, or to pseudoephedrine, and even natural ephedra, an herb used in many diet and energy supplements. In my case, for example, I used to be able to take a Sudafed without a problem. Now, I find I can only take half a capsule without developing some heart palpitations. And I *really* have to be careful not to take it with a caffeinated beverage, or I definitely have an hour of palpitations. I can take other cold products and antihistamines, for example, without a problem. I typically will choose cold medicines that don't include pseudoephedrine.

My recommendation? Talk to your doctor about these products before you try them, and if you get the go-ahead, try a much smaller dose than usual, see if it affects you, and if you feel okay, try working your way up to the normal dose.

What about Thyroid Hormone and Estrogen?

Taking estrogen in any form, whether as hormone replacement therapy, or in birth control pills, can affect thyroid test results.

For example, some women taking estrogen may need to take more thyroid replacement hormone. The hormone replacement therapies (such as Estrace, Estraderm, Premarin, Prempro, Estradiol, and various forms of the Pill) increase a particular protein that binds thyroid hormone to it, making the thyroid hormone partially inactive. Thyroid tests can end up showing falsely increased total T-4 levels. For women without thyroids in particular, this can increase the dosage requirement slightly, as there is no thyroid to compensate. Being on thyroid hormone replacement certainly does not mean you shouldn't take estrogen or birth control pills prescribed by your doctor. However, after beginning any estrogen therapy, you should have thyroid tests run six to eight weeks later to see if the addition of estrogen means you'll need a thyroid dosage adjustment. Also, be sure the doctor prescribing the Pill or estrogen replacement is aware that you're on thyroid hormone.

Interactions with Antidepressants and Thyroid Hormone

Use of tricyclic antidepressants such as doxepin, amitriptyline, desipramine, and impramine—some brand names include Adapin, Elavil, Norpramin, and Tofranil—at the same time as thyroid hormones may increase the effects of both drugs and may *accelerate the effects of the antidepressant.* Be sure your doctor knows you are on one before prescribing the other.

Also, researchers have found that taking thyroid hormone replacement while taking the popular antidepressant sertraline—(Zoloft)—can cause a *decrease in the effectiveness of the thyroid hormone replacement.* This same effect has also been seen in patients receiving other selective serotonin-reuptake inhibitors such as paroxetine (Paxil) and fluoxetine (Prozac).

If you are on an antidepressant or thyroid hormone and your doctor wants to prescribe the other, be sure to discuss these issues.

Other Drug Interactions

A number of other drugs interact with thyroid hormone or affect thyroid function.

- *Insulin*—Thyroid hormone can reduce the effectiveness of insulin and the similar drugs for diabetes. Be sure your doctor knows you are on one before prescribing the other.

- *Cholesterol-Lowering Drugs Cholestyramine or Colestipol*— These drugs—known by brand names such as Colestrol, Questran,

Colestid—bind thyroid hormones. A minimum of *four to five hours* should elapse between taking these drugs and thyroid hormones.

• *Anticoagulants ("Blood Thinners")*—Anticoagulant drugs like Warfarin, Coumadin, or Heparin can sometimes become stronger in the system when thyroid hormone is added to the mix. Mention it to your doctor if you are on one or the other.

• *Corticosteroids/Adrenocorticosteroids*—Brands include Cortisone, Cortistab, and Cortone. These drugs suppress TSH and can block conversion of T4 to T3 in some people.

• *Amiodarone HCL*—The heart drug known by the brand name Cordarone can cause hypothyroidism or hyperthyroidism and interfere with T4 metabolism. People taking Cordarone should be monitored periodically for thyroid changes.

• *Ketamine*—Some people have elevated blood pressure and a racing heartbeat when they've taken levothyroxine sodium and the anesthetic ketamine at the same time.

• *Maprotiline*—This antidepressant can increase a risk of cardiac arrhythmias when taken with thyroid hormone products.

• *Theophylline*—This drug for asthma and respiratory diseases may not clear out of the body as quickly when someone is hypothyroid, but usually clears normally when the thyroid is in the normal range.

• *Lithium*—Lithium is known to actually create hypothyroidism by blocking secretion of T4 and T3. People taking lithium should be monitored periodically for thyroid changes.

• *Phenytoin*—This anticonvulsant, a brand of which is Dilantin, may accelerate levothyroxine metabolism, and tests may show decreased total T4 levels.

• *Carbamazepine*—This anticonvulsant pain medicine, a brand of which is Tegretol, may accelerate levothyroxine metabolism, and tests may show decreased total T4 levels.

• *Rifampin*—This antituberculosis agent may accelerate levothyroxine metabolism, and tests may show decreased total T4 levels.

What About "Goitrogenic" Foods?

Goitrogens are products and foods that promote formation of goiters. They can act like antithyroid drugs in disabling the thyroid and cause hypothyroidism. Specifically, goitrogens have some ability to inhibit the body's ability to use iodine, block the process by which iodine becomes the thyroid hormones T4 and T3, inhibit the actual secretion of thyroid hormone, and disrupt the peripheral conversion of T4 to T3.

If you are hypothyroid due to thyroidectomy, you don't have to be particularly concerned about goitrogens. If you still have a thyroid, however, you need to be more concerned about goitrogens, and be careful not to eat them uncooked in large quantities. Some experts believe that the enzymes involved in the formation of goitrogenic materials in plants can be destroyed by cooking, so thorough cooking may minimize some or most goitrogenic potential. Eating reasonable amounts of goitrogenic foods, raw or cooked, is probably not a problem for most people.

What foods are goitrogens? Brussels sprouts, rutabaga, turnips, kohlrabi, radishes, cauliflower, African cassava, millet, babassu (a palm-tree coconut fruit popular in Brazil and Africa) cabbage, kale, and soy products are all considered goitrogenic.

Seasonal Variations in Thyroid Hormone Requirements

One little-known issue for thyroid patients in terms of their dosage of thyroid hormone is the seasonal variation in thyroid function.

There haven't been enough studies that evaluate exactly how the dosage requirements fluctuate and how they should be adjusted to take seasonal changes into account. Research shows, however, that TSH naturally rises during colder months and drops to low normal or even hyperthyroid levels in the warmest months. Some doctors will adjust for this by prescribing slightly increased dosages during colder months and reducing dosage during warm periods. Most, however, are not aware of this seasonal fluctuation, and patients suffer worsening hypothyroidism symptoms during cold winter months, and hyperthyroidism symptoms during warmer months due to slight overdosage.

This seasonal fluctuation becomes more pronounced in older people and in particularly cold climates. To maintain optimal wellness, seasonal variation in TSH should be taken into consideration when evaluating the adequacy of a levothyroxine replacement dose. Patients should insist on having more than an annual blood test. Instead, twice-yearly tests, at minimum during winter and summer months, should help assess the fluctuation, so that an adequate general replacement dosage and modification for seasonal change can be determined.

How Long Will It Really Take to Feel Better?

Once you're diagnosed and begin thyroid hormone replacement, the most obvious question is how long will it take until you feel better.

Many doctors and endocrinologists tell patients that it might take two weeks to start feeling better. Some people actually do feel well as early as two weeks after starting thyroid hormone replacement . . . but not most people.

For example, it took about four months for me to *start* feeling human again as my TSH crept down from a high of 15, plus several more months after that to tweak and get dosages even better in range.

Think of it this way. It takes months or years not a few weeks— for your body to get hypothyroid in the first place. It's not a magic pill like an aspirin that takes away a headache in minutes, unfortunately. When you start taking a T4-only medication like Synthroid, it takes two weeks for it to be reflected in your TSH levels. Then, your body needs to absorb, use and apply it, healing things that have gone awry.

Knowing that I wasn't expected to feel perfect again right away was comforting in its own way. I wanted to feel better quickly, but

I also had hope that I would continue to improve over time. I think having realistic expectations can make you feel better, even if you still don't feel well physically.

Some say that autoimmune diseases strike "Type A" personalities more often. We want to control, to do more and more and more, go faster, higher, better, and this condition lays us low and forces us to give up control. Infuriating! The one thing I really learned was how patience is essential. I'm *not* good at that. But I had to try, and you do, too.

While waiting for your thyroid hormone replacement to kick into action, do other things for yourself as much as possible. Try to get extra rest. Get a massage, or visit an acupuncture session for energy. Take a yoga or T'ai Chi class. Get a temporary membership at a health club, and do some gentle exercising. Treat yourself, pamper yourself, and figure you're helping your recuperation, helping your body to heal as you're on your way to living well.

PART II

CHALLENGES AND ALTERNATIVES

CHAPTER 6

Challenges in Getting Diagnosed and Treated

Doubt whom you will, but never yourself.
BOVEE

Many of you have a difficult time getting a diagnosis of hypothyroidism, despite clear signs of the condition. You may have a doctor who is reluctant to test, or one who is too conservative in interpreting lab ranges, or you may face other issues that delay diagnosis. Even getting your doctor to the most basic step, the TSH test, can be a challenge for some.

Because a proper diagnosis is absolutely essential in order to live well, it's important to look at the diagnostic and treatment challenges you might encounter, and how to successfully resolve them.

A TENDENCY NOT TO TRUST
YOUR OWN INSTINCTS

Many people have told me that, retrospectively, they realize something was wrong but didn't act on it or mention it to the doctor early enough. Some people assumed weight gain was due to a change in diet, or presumed their exhaustion was due to excess obligations.

Geri, a health writer and producer in NY, was diagnosed as hypothyroid during a routine physical, but looking back, realized that she had the signs of hypothyroidism for a number of years:

At the time I was diagnosed, I didn't think I had any symptoms. But in retrospect, I had started feeling *very* cold and generally sluggish and sickly for about two months before I was diagnosed. I chalked it up to general fatigue, overwork, wintertime blues, approaching thirty. Looking farther back, I think my thyroid started to go about five years ago. At that time, I stopped getting my period for twenty months and gained weight.

If you suspect or believe something's wrong, chances are you may be right. Trust your intuition, and go to the doctor sooner rather than later.

YOUR DOCTOR'S REFUSAL TO TEST YOUR THYROID

Some doctors are resistant to your request for a thyroid test. Sometimes, they are protecting their ego and sense of superiority, and in other cases, they may be reacting to management measures that discourage costly medical tests.

One patient, D.J., faced a reluctant doctor:

I had asked for a thyroid test no less than three times over the course of nine months and was given some other test instead. She finally agreed grudgingly to a thyroid test. Imagine "our" surprise to find out my hunch was correct all along! My TSH was so high, the lab thought their analysis machine was broken!

After getting her diagnosis, D.J. found a new doctor who does not feel threatened by patients who take an active role in their health care.

Charl, a medical professional in the military, went to her military doctor to request that her thyroid be checked:

I was countered with, "Now Major, not everyone who is overweight is hypothyroid (as he checked my neck manually). Besides, who is the doctor here?!" I asked if a blood test needed to be conducted to determine whether or not my thyroid was faulty. "Do you think you can tell me my job?! Your thyroid is normal. I just checked your neck!!!" I decided it was time to seek the advice of a civilian physician. She ordered a plethora of tests and discovered that I have Hashimoto's thyroiditis.

Some doctors discourage testing because they are in an HMO or managed care environment where their rating, reputation, or even incomes are affected by the number of tests they order. According to Dr. John Lowe:

> Managed care companies provide incentives to physicians for not ordering laboratory tests, not treating patients, and not referring them to specialists. So physicians working for these companies may decline to order laboratory tests so that their income will be higher.

When faced with a doctor who refuses to test your thyroid, the best option is to find another doctor, even if you have to pay for it yourself. But if you have no options, here are a few tips:

• Be persistent. Ask for a thyroid test. Show the doctor articles about hypothyroidism that reflect your symptoms, even if he or she won't read them. Ask again and again.
• Bring your Hypothyroidism Checklist to an appointment, and ask that it be included in your medical chart after the doctor signs, dates it, and indicates that he or she has read the checklist and discussed it with you. Make sure you get a signed and dated copy for yourself. Send a copy to the HMO's or insurance company's ombudsman or consumer liaison, along with your request that testing be approved.
• Write a simple letter that states that for the reasons listed, you have specifically requested that you be tested for thyroid disease, and that this doctor has refused. Insist that the doctor sign it, and place a copy in your charts, and give you a copy. (You can then send this copy to the HMO to argue for a referral to another doctor or an endocrinologist, if needed.)

I've frequently suggested these ideas to people who write to me at the Web site, and they often work. Most doctors will order the test rather than officially document their decision to refuse a patient's request. Apparently, the concerns over malpractice or mismanagement charges made by patients override their reluctance to test. It may seem ridiculous that you have to fight to get standard medical tests and treatment, but it's your health that is at stake, so keep fighting.

SYMPTOM-BY-SYMPTOM DIAGNOSIS MISSES THE BIG PICTURE

Some people go in to see the doctor over the course of months or years with symptom after symptom of hypothyroidism. The doctor treats each individual condition—cholesterol drugs for elevated cholesterol, antidepressants for depression, appetite suppressants for weight gain—but doesn't step back, look at the big picture, and say, "Aha, a classic textbook list of hypothyroidism symptoms. Maybe I should run a thyroid test."

LuAnn's experiences are a good example of what many people go through. She started with swollen eyes, then developed pins and needles in her legs, painful leg muscles, slurred speech, a thick tongue, and swollen face. At each step of the way, her doctor said the problems were allergies, sinus problems, vitamin deficiencies, and so on. Even LuAnn's mother and husband were wondering if something was going on with LuAnn's thyroid, and when asked, the doctor said she didn't think so. Finally, after many months, the doctor agreed to test LuAnn's thyroid:

> On Friday evening I received a call from our clinic. It was the doctor on call that night. She said that my blood work results had just come in and that she was very worried and needed to get me on some medication immediately. My heart was pounding, and I think I started sobbing on the phone, just because someone was saying that, yes, there is actually something wrong with you! She said that my T4 was not even borderline. It was 0.4. And she had never seen a higher TSH, which was 460.

In this case, again, when your instincts and even other people are telling you that there's a thyroid problem, you may have to try another doctor and get a second opinion to break out of the symptom-by-symptom diagnosis rut. The Hypothyroidism Checklist can also help in presenting to your doctor a comprehensive overview of all your possible symptoms and how they fit together into a possible diagnosis worth investigating.

MISDIAGNOSIS AS DEPRESSION, STRESS, OR PMS—AND GENDER BIAS

The demonstrated relationship between depression and hypothyroidism is discussed in greater depth in chapter 10. But at the diagnostic stage, it's important to note that because depression is more common than hypothyroidism, you are more likely to initially walk away with a diagnosis of depression than with a thyroid test. Some researchers estimate that as much as 15 percent or more of people with a diagnosis of depression are *actually* suffering from undiagnosed hypothyroidism.

Many forward-thinking doctors believe that a thyroid test should *always* be performed to rule out thyroid disease as a cause of depression. Kate Lemmerman, M.D., says:

> Even if someone comes in complaining specifically of depression, I believe they need to have a thorough evaluation done, including, but not limited to, thyroid testing, before being prescribed an antidepressant.

Women face a particular version of this misdiagnosis. Some doctors don't take women's health complaints as seriously as they take those from men. This type of doctor assumes that women are more emotional or even sometimes "hysterical" and are overstating their symptoms or the severity of their symptoms. Because hypothyroidism affects women far more than men, this bias against women can also explain in part why some doctors fail to make a proper diagnosis.

There's often an assumption that changes in weight, mood, and energy—also frequently the symptoms of hypothyroidism—are merely a result of normal cyclical changes in a woman's "hormonal" status. It's true that weight, mood, and energy can change due to the hormonal system, but the thyroid is part of that system too, not just estrogen.

Having your symptoms overlooked or ignored because you are a woman is particularly frustrating. Dr. Kate Lemmerman explains why this phenomenon still occurs with some doctors:

> I believe that when women complain of weight gain, fatigue, dry skin, constipation, and other complaints classic for hypothyroidism it is often thought that these complaints are psychological . . . and they are prescribed an antidepressant without first checking to see if there is an organic reason for their complaints. I think we still view women as "the weaker sex" and so more easily write off their symptoms without adequately evaluating them.

While thyroid problems strike women five to seven times more often, there are still many men who develop hypothyroidism. Because hypothyroidism is less common in men, and because men are less likely to mention some of the symptoms to their doctors, getting a diagnosis can become particularly difficult for men as well.

Lee, a man in his mid-forties, spent most of his adulthood plagued by depression, lethargy, dry skin, and incredibly cold fingers. Typical thyroid symptoms, but like many men, he was less likely than a woman to be tested for an underactive thyroid. Eventually, the doctor tested him because of extremely high and unresponsive cholesterol levels above 300:

> I was going to refuse the test. That he is the first doctor to look at my description of my life and suggest that thyroid tests were needed sort of shocks me. I am overjoyed that some of the complaints I have can be dealt with so effectively for the first time.

Tom had to go through many months of complaints and a misdiagnosis of depression before he was able to get a diagnosis:

> Being a man, I have found it hard to get doctors to listen, possibly worse, because they want to categorize hypothyroidism as a "woman's disease." I have tried to explain to them that I am not trying to say

I am having menstrual problems, I am not asking for a mammogram, I am asking for you to treat my thyroid, a piece of anatomy that, the last time I checked, is shared by men and woman alike. I often wonder how many men are out there either too proud and macho to realize they are sick, or are being misdiagnosed as being "depressed" and being put on drugs that do not help the problem.

Again, if you suspect that you're being written off as depressed or "hormonal"—when the real issue is an underlying thyroid condition—be persistent and repeatedly ask for thyroid testing. Insist that a copy of your Hypothyroidism Checklist or a letter indicating your doctor's refusal to test you be signed and included in your medical chart. Also, remember that the more businesslike and calm you can be, the more likely you will be able to make your case to the doctor. It might be hard, and it might seem unfair or even ridiculous that you have to "convince" your doctor to do what's right, but let's get beyond what's right or fair, and move on to what will result in your wellness.

THE DIAGNOSTIC "TYRANNY OF THE TSH"

Dr. John Lowe refers to the exclusive use of the TSH test to diagnose and manage hypothyroidism as "the tyranny of the TSH." And Dr. Lowe is right—the TSH test can be a tyrant.

In the past, thyroid disease was diagnosed and managed using a combination of blood tests, medical history, examination, and discussion of symptoms. Some doctors also used the basal body temperature test. Today, however, you'll find it difficult to convince many conventional doctors to do more than a TSH test in order to diagnose or manage your hypothyroidism. They've seemingly abandoned generations of medical knowledge and diagnostic tools, preferring to rely on one result—the TSH test—that often has nothing to do with how patients actually feel. In this purely conventional view of health, a normal TSH value—or what they refer to as being euthyroid—is equal to thyroid health.

This rigid interpretation of the TSH test is sometimes even carried to the extreme. Some doctors actually refuse to consider treatment for a patient who has hypothyroidism symptoms, a family history, and a TSH of 4.9 TSH—when over 5 is considered hypothyroid. The same doctors will diagnose hypothyroidism and prescribe treatment for a TSH of 5.1. Symptoms you have at 5.1 will be attributed to your hypothyroidism, but once TSH levels are under 5, your doctor may say that the same symptoms are now unrelated to your thyroid. It doesn't make much sense.

Kate Lemmerman, M.D. shared this overview of medical school education on hypothyroidism:

> When I was in medical school we covered the pathology of hypothyroidism very well. But we often failed to consider the human impact of the disease and how best to deal with that. Therefore, if someone's TSH normalized then our treatment was successful. If they still felt fatigued, then perhaps it was depression or something "they would just have to learn to live with." And if someone's TSH was "within normal limits" but they had complaints that seemed like hypothyroidism, we were not taught to think that perhaps the range of "normal limits" may not be the ideal levels for proper functioning in that person.

The idea that "normal is normal is normal" and that as long as you fall somewhere in the normal range you are properly diagnosed and/or adequately treated is slowing falling by the wayside. Anecdotal evidence exists that "normal" for most people without thyroid disease may, in fact, be under a TSH of 2. My endocrinologist and some others, for example, firmly believe that most women thyroid patients feel best in the 1 to 2 TSH range, and that above that level, there's greater difficulty in getting pregnant, avoiding miscarriage, losing weight, and getting rid of other symptoms. I've also heard from various medical professionals, including lab technicians, who have indicated that anecdotally, they find that the average TSH for people who are not suffering from thyroid disease was around 1. It was not a wide distribution from .5 to 5, but instead concentrated more tightly around a TSH of 1.

More than just anecdotal evidence also exists showing that "normal" may actually be in the lower end of the range. According to A. P. Weetman, a professor of medicine at the University of Sheffield, writing in the respected *British Medical Journal*:

. . . thyroid-stimulating hormone (TSH) concentrations above 2 mU/ l reflect a disturbance of the thyroid-pituitary axis, values above the upper level of the typical reference range (4.5 mU/l) are highly significant departures from normal rather than one tail of the normal distribution.

Weetman also found that a TSH level greater than 2 was associated with an increased risk of future hypothyroidism. He theorizes that thyroid disease may be so common that many "abnormal" people who are on their way to becoming fully hypothyroid are included in the "normal" reference values. This suggests that the normal TSH for people who are not now and never will become hypothyroid may well be under 2.

If you've had a TSH test and been told you're normal, there's more fact-finding you need to do. First, do not accept "you're in the normal range" as a report of your results. Ask for your specific numbers and the lab's normal ranges. Better yet, ask for a photocopy of the test results page, so you can keep it in your own file.

If you have specifically requested the numbers and your doctor refuses to tell you, insisting "it's normal," or "you don't need to know the numbers," or "leave the doctoring to me," this is a *major* warning that you need another doctor. There is absolutely no valid reason for a doctor to refuse to share your lab results. If the doctor refuses, then it's due to an overinflated ego or an assumption that you deserve no role in your own health care, good reasons to look for another doctor. As Dr. Susan Osborne emphasizes: "You pay for the lab work, you have an *absolute* right to know your numbers."

You might also want to check your health records to see if you've ever had your thyroid tested in the past. If the test occurred *before* you started to develop thyroid symptoms, you may have a true picture of what *your* normal TSH value is. Sometimes, being able to see a rise from a lower normal TSH level to high-normal or slightly above normal is enough for your doctor to consider diagnosing hypothyroidism.

If you are one of the people who is functionally hypothyroid with a normal or high-normal TSH level, you may need additional tests—such as the antibodies test, TRH test, or T3 and Reverse T3 tests—to get a true diagnosis of your hypothyroidism. If your doctor is willing to test for TSH and nothing else, you're probably not going to have much luck getting any further than this without changing doctors. In particular, if you want to pursue tests like Reverse T3 or TRH, you'll probably need to find a more open-minded holistic doctor or practitioner.

If you are already under treatment for hypothyroidism, and don't feel well in the middle- or high-normal range, you should also discuss targeting a lower TSH level with your doctor. Some doctors are reluctant to target lower TSH levels because they are concerned that lower TSH levels can increase the risk of osteoporosis. This is a very controversial issue, one discussed in greater depth in chapter 14. Right now, it's important that you know, however, that there are research findings on *both* sides of the osteoporasis issue. Some studies find there is no increased risk or the increased risk is not statistically significant. Others find that the risk is real. What we do know is that doctors who tell you that taking too much thyroid hormone will *definitely* increase your risk of osteoporosis are not telling you the whole story.

DOCTORS RELUCTANT TO TREAT
BORDERLINE HYPOTHYROIDISM

One self-proclaimed thyroid expert—an internist I consulted for a second opinion on my hypothyroidism—told me that as far as he was concerned a patient can't possibly have symptoms at supposedly mild levels of hypothyroidism, such as a TSH level of 6 or 8 or 10.

He was adamant about this, insisting that no one would feel any symptoms until TSH went well above 10. Speaking as someone who can tell by my symptoms the difference between a TSH of 2 and 5, I didn't go back to him for any more second opinions because he's dead wrong. Many people have symptoms at even normal or high-normal TSH levels, much less levels that are actually hypothyroid by lab standards.

Diann experienced problems when she discovered that her doctor felt her TSH level was barely worth treating:

> The doctor's office minimized my symptoms to the point of casually
> leaving a message on my voice mail that "your tests are a little high,"

when indeed the TSH level was 12. I had to retrieve my medical records to find this out. No wonder I felt like I was losing my personality, abilities, spunk, and ME. Did the internist make an effort to empathize or consult me personally?? NO! Seemingly, I wasn't suffering in his "book."

Toy Lin also suffered with hypothyroidism needlessly for years because she didn't ask about the specific numbers, and her doctor apparently didn't believe that borderline hypothyroidism deserved treatment:

I'm so mad!! The last three or four years I've been on a downhill slide. I told the endocrinologist I had all these symptoms. He ignored me. I just got copies of my blood tests and see that the tests showed my TSH went from 1.6 in 1994 to 6.31 in 1996. The lab marked 6.31 as being high. The endo told me I was fine, I was normal. I have lost all this time, been a couch potato since then, because he ignored how I felt.

As Toy Lin's experience shows, it's very important to know your TSH numbers and pursue treatment when warranted.

DOCTORS WHO WON'T TREAT HIGH ANTIBODY LEVELS

It is not uncommon to test positive for thyroid antibodies yet have a normal TSH. The combination of antibodies and hypothyroidism symptoms usually means your thyroid is in the process of autoimmune failure. Not failed to the extent that it even registers as an elevated TSH level, but in the process of failing.

Many doctors, however, believe that as long as TSH is normal, testing positive for thyroid antibodies is *not* sufficient reason to prescribe thyroid hormone, even when you are plagued by the symptoms of hypothyroidism.

There are, however, some conventional doctors, and even more nonconventional doctors and health practitioners, who believe that the presence of thyroid antibodies, along with symptoms of hypo-thyroidism, warrant treatment.

One such practitioner is Elizabeth Vliet, M.D., a doctor who runs HER Place®, women's health clinics in Tucson, Arizona, and Dallas/Fort Worth, Texas. Dr. Vliet is also author of one of my favorite health books, *Screaming to be Heard: Hormonal Connections Women Suspect . . . and Doctors Ignore*. Dr. Vliet believes that symptoms, along with elevated thyroid antibodies and normal TSH, may be a reason for treatment with thyroid hormone. In her book, Dr. Vliet writes:

> The problem I have found is that too often women are told their thyroid is normal without having the complete thyroid tests done. Of course, what most people, and many physicians, don't realize is that . . . a "normal range" on a laboratory report is just that: a range. A given person may require higher or lower levels to feel well and to function optimally. I think we must look at the lab results along with the clinical picture described by the patient. . . . I have a series of more than a hundred patients, all but two are women, who had a normal TSH and turned out to have significantly elevated thyroid antibodies that meant they needed thyroid medication in order to feel normal . . . a woman may experience the symptoms of disease months to years before TSH goes up. . . .

Dr. Vliet's thoughtful ideas and innovative approaches are supported by research that has found that people may experience thyroid-related symptoms, such as fatigue and depression, before thyroid levels become abnormal. Interestingly, like Dr. Vliet, these same researchers found that people with elevated thyroid antibodies, but normal TSH range, responded favorably, both physically and emotionally, to low-dose thyroid hormone treatment. At the same time, taking the thyroid hormone did not induce hyperthyroidism or create any side effects.

Thyroid antibodies are also proven to affect fertility and the ability to maintain a pregnancy. For example, the risk of miscarriage can be as much as double for women who have antithyroid antibodies as in those who do not.

Later in this chapter you'll find more guidance on how to find the kind of doctor who will treat you for high thyroid antibodies if you have hypothyroidism symptoms.

DOCTORS WHO DON'T USE THE TRH TEST

The TRH test is still used by some open-minded doctors to measure the thyroid's actual responsiveness and to uncover resistance to thyroid hormone, including peripheral resistance problems. Most mainstream doctors believe that the TRH test is no longer useful or necessary in diagnosing hypothyroidism given the so-called accuracy of the TSH test. I've heard from patients and their doctors who couldn't find labs where they could even conduct a TRH test, it is considered so uncommon.

Dr. John Lowe believes that part of the difficulty in finding a doctor to do a TRH stimulation test is that some researchers believe that pituitary-based hypothyroidism can be diagnosed with the usual laboratory thyroid function tests. They say if the patient has a low TSH and a low T4 level, the function of the pituitary gland is impaired because a low T4 level should increase the TSH level. Says Dr. Lowe:

> We studied this question and found that we were not able to predict which patients would be found to have impaired pituitary function (according to the TRH stimulation test) based on the TSH and T4 levels. In other words, there was no relationship between impaired pituitary function, according to the TRH stimulation test, and TSH and T4 levels. Our analysis indicates that patients with central hypothyroidism are likely to go undiagnosed unless they have a TRH stimulation test.

Many people have asked their doctors for TRH tests, only to be told that there's nowhere to get such a test in their area, or that they have no idea how to conduct one. Dr. Lowe, who interprets TRH test results regularly in his practice, offers these recommendations:

> One option is for patients to call different doctors' offices until they find one who performs the TRH stimulation test. I would suggest

starting with holistic physicians. Many of these practitioners question the mandates of conventional medicine and provide rational testing and treatment despite the mandates. If a patient has a cooperative physician who is willing to learn to do the test, the physician can obtain the supplies and publications needed from the company that markets them.

Doctors who are interested in supplies for the TRH test can obtain injectable 500 microgram boluses of Thyrel (TRH) by contacting Ferring Laboratories, 400 Rella Blvd., Ste 201, Suffern, NY 10901 Tel. (914) 368-7916 FAX (914) 368-1193. Dr. Lowe also recommends that patients and physicians obtain a copy of his paper, "Thyroid Status of 38 Fibromyalgia Patients: Implications for the Etiology of Fibromyalgia," which was published in *The Clinical Bulletin of Myofascial Therapy*, vol. 2, no.1, pp.47-64, 1997. The article includes extensive information on the interpretation of the TRH stimulation tests.

DOCTORS WHO DON'T RECOGNIZE THYROID HORMONE CONVERSION AND RESISTANCE PROBLEMS

When you get into the realm of thyroid "conversion," you really start losing most conventional doctors. This is the area of thyroid physiology and treatment that is least understood by conventional medicine, and where most of the alternative thyroid diagnostic and treatment protocols are finding success.

To understand conversion problems, let's take another look at how the thyroid operates. The healthy thyroid produces T4 and T3. Depending on what book you read, the percentage is anywhere from 80 to 95 percent T4, and 5 to 20 percent T3. Since T3 is the biologically active hormone, T4 is converted to T3 for use at the cellular level.

We know that the normal process of T4 to T3 conversion can, to some extent, be temporarily inhibited by various stress on the body, illness, fasting, pregnancy, high levels of stress hormones in the body (cortisol), and other factors.

Here is where things get more controversial. Most conventional doctors feel that the body almost always converts the T4 to the T3 at levels appropriate for ongoing functioning. Therefore, even if you've had your thyroid removed, or have an underfunctioning thyroid, you only need T4, not additional T3. This is the argument you'll hear from most doctors and endocrinologists.

Some doctors believe that the conversion process may be impaired for some people. They feel that T4 may not properly convert to T3, leaving T3 levels too low. Or T4 is not properly converting to T3 at the cellular level, leaving cells hypothyroid and starving for thyroid hormone, despite normal blood test values.

In some cases, the problem may not even be conversion, but in the cell's ability to even *use* the thyroid hormone. John Lowe refers to it as peripheral thyroid hormone resistance. According to Dr. Susan Osborne, some patients on conventional thyroid drugs will have normal TSH levels but still suffer from hypothyroidism and its symptoms because they have antibodies to the enzyme that *converts* T4 to T3, making insufficient amounts of T3 available to the cells.

In these cases, when a deficiency in T3 is suspected, innovative practitioners are willing to treat patients with T3. These doctors prescribe Cytomel or time-released T3 to be added to a regimen of levothyroxine. In some cases, they prefer the combination synthetic T4/T3 drug Thyrolar or one of the natural thyroid products that contains T4 and T3.

It's medical fact that in times of physical stress the body converts T4 to an inactive form of T3 known as Reverse T3. One former doctor theorized that the body can get "stuck" in this mode, leaving cells deficient in thyroid hormone and hypothyroid, despite normal blood test values. This theory, known as "Wilson's Syndrome," is named after Denis Wilson, formerly a licensed physician, who initially described this process and claimed that it is the cause of numerous health problems. Wilson believes that a major stress—such as childbirth, divorce, surgery, accident, or ongoing family/work pressure—slows the body down as a coping mechanism. The body temperature can drop as a response, which is normal. Wilson's theory says that sometimes the temperature remains low even after the stress has passed.

A diagnosis of Wilson's Syndrome includes symptoms, as well as body temperature, taken using a Mercury thermometer, every three hours, three times a day, starting three hours after waking, for several days (but excluding the period three days before menstruation for women, as temperatures rise during that time.) If you woke at 7 a.m., then you'd take the temperature again at 10 a.m., 1 p.m., and 4 p.m. Add the temperatures together each day, and divide by three, to get an average. If the average is less than 98.6, Wilson's Syndrome proponents claim that you might have the problem. The Wilson's Syndrome protocol uses T3 to help resolve this T3 imbalance.

It's my belief that "Wilson's Syndrome" should be renamed to something neutral and less likely to incur the ire of doctors. To be honest, Wilson has a questionable reputation. He has a history of several out-of-court settlements on a number of different complaints and charges. Wilson's Web site claims his legal problems have nothing to do with negligence or the protocol itself. Wilson, however, has apparently not gone back to active medical practice, instead launching his for-profit "Wilson's Syndrome Foundation," selling costly books, tapes, and informational binders describing his protocol and how it solves everything from excess weight to skin problems to ongoing fatigue.

I am suspicious of anyone who believes that the answer to a whole list of problems just happens to be the thing he sells. But what Wilson describes is not outlandish. Little is known about the role of T3 and Reverse T3 in relieving patient's symptoms. Reverse T3 problems may in fact be one key to the puzzle of truly resolving hypothyroidism.

Mention conversion problem, Reverse T3 or Wilson's Syndrome to many conventional doctors and you'll get a lecture about quack medicine, pseudoscience, and the dangers of the Internet, among other diatribes. You may be told you can't possibly have Wilson's Disease (a rare inability to process copper that has nothing to do with your thyroid). And if you mention "resistance," you'll come up against the difference between peripheral resistance and general resistance. Peripheral resistance refers to the ability to convert T4 to T3 in organs and cells, and according to some doctors, may be a fairly common problem. "Generalized" resistance to thyroid hormone (RTH) is a very rare genetic disorder. When people suggest to their doctors, "Maybe I am resistant to thyroid hormone," doctors are usually quick to dismiss this, assuming that you mean you think you have RTH, which would be highly unlikely for the vast majority of the population.

At worst, you might encounter hostility or even be "fired" by your doctor, the situation in which one thyroid patient, Tom, found himself:

> I tried very hard to get the doctor to listen to me and he rolled his eyes and said "I don't care what crap you heard on the Internet." I was just trying to ask what I felt were educated questions based on what I have read, but I got accused by the doctor of trying to "tell me how to do my job." Then he did what I still can't believe. He actually had the gall to tell me, "You're not welcome here anymore. Take your labs and your questions and comments and find another doctor. I don't want to see you again telling me how to do my job . . . if you ask me you just have a depression problem that maybe you should get looked at." I told him his bedside manner sucked, that all I was trying to do is be an advocate for myself and be involved in my own treatment.

Ultimately, getting "fired" by his doctor was the best thing that ever happened to Tom because he went on to find a doctor that *did* diagnose his hypothyroidism, and Tom is finally feeling much better.

For more in-depth discussion of several innovative philosophies and research findings regarding T3, see chapter 8. If you want to pursue a diagnosis of, or treatment for, conversion problems, you might try contacting some holistic or alternative doctors and asking in advance if they recognize and treat these types of problems.

FINDING THE RIGHT DOCTOR

In some cases, the key to getting the right diagnosis and treatment is finding a new doctor, not always an easy proposition.

When it comes to treating hypothyroidism, my bias is toward more holistic, alternative practitioners. My regular family doctor is a holistic M.D., who practices with several osteopathic physicians. She is also trained in acupuncture and osteopathy. My doctor listens, cares, is interested in learning more every day, is up on the latest developments, and never rushes, never makes me feel that I'm wasting her time, and never discards what patients think or feel in her overall process of diagnosis. And to be fair, on the downside, she is very popular and thus not always easy to get in to see, usually makes you wait, is expensive, and not on any health insurance plans. I do periodically check in with a conventional endocrinologist, but her main contribution to my health has been the idea that a lower TSH of 1 to 2 is, in fact, optimal for many women in order to avoid symptoms, feel well, and maintain normal fertility and pregnancy.

I tend to favor more holistic practitioners for hypothyroidism because it's a particularly tricky condition for conventional medicine. If you're one of the people with elevated TSH who responds perfectly to levothyroxine, conventional doctoring can work well for you. For everyone else, there are no clear models for conventional doctors to follow. Philosophically, they are coming out of an educational system that emphasizes what are known as "bugs and drugs"—doctors' lingo for illnesses and the drugs used to treat them. In the short time that their medical education involves hypothyroidism, conventional medical school graduates learn that hypothyroidism is a simple, easily treated "bug" that is diagnosed using the TSH test results and treated with the "drug" thyroid hormone. With endocrinology programs at most major medical schools beholden in part to the financial support of pharmaceutical companies, it's not likely that anything other than the TSH test/levothyroxine treatment approach will be taught for a long time to come.

When you look at the curriculum and training offered in osteopathic medical schools or specialized training in holistic, alternative or complementary medicine, you'll see more of a focus on the sorts of interrelationships found in hypothyroidism. Doctors trained in these schools and approaches will usually have a greater openness to using the full wealth of diagnostic options—patient symptoms, basal body temperature, antibodies testing, TRH tests, and more. These doctors, whether M.D.s or D.O.s, are more likely to be aware of alternative thyroid drugs or supplemental alternative and complementary treatments for hypothyroidism. They learn more about the importance of listening in diagnosis, the value of many diagnostic tools, and the "holistic" aspect of health.

Despite my bias, I have to say that there are many fine, caring, wonderful conventional doctors. And there are holistic doctors and osteopaths who are narrow-minded or whose main objective is to sell you expensive vitamins, potions, and tinctures, and subject you to expensive—and even wacky—tests that put money in their pockets. So your job is to sort through and find the best—the most honest—doctors, whatever initials they have after their names, for you and your health.

As far as the right doctor, take a look at the different types of doctors you might see for your hypothyroidism, and evaluate their strengths and weaknesses. I'm going to generalize here, so there are always going to be wonderful doctors who break every mold and defy every stereotype. These guidelines might help, however, in making some decisions regarding your treatment.

Endocrinologists

An endocrinologist specializes in diseases of the endocrine system. Endocrinologists typically have the initials F.A.C.E. after their names, standing for Fellow of the American College of Endocrinology. The two main issues endocrinologists deal with are diabetes and thyroid problems. Some endocrinologists, however, have subspecialties like reproductive endocrinology (fertility), nuclear medicine, growth disorders, or osteoporosis. To be honest, the big issue with endocrinologists is finding one who thinks thyroid disease is interesting. Many of them focus almost exclusively on diabetes and treat thyroid problems as a sideline. Almost 16 million Americans have diabetes, but that is more than the estimated 13 million with thyroid disease. Diabetes typically has more serious side-effects and complications, and there are more medicines to play with, so it attracts more interest.

Endocrinologists are often characterized as "numbers-lovers," preferring to read lab charts and TSH levels over patient interaction or creative problem-solving. Often, there isn't much difference between one endocrinologist and another. Unless they're one of the rare breed who are truly open to new information or they have some unconventional solutions, they're fairly interchangeable. All endocrinologists can read a TSH chart and write Synthroid prescriptions. What differentiates some endocrinologists from the rest, frankly, is kindness, personality, sympathy, responsiveness, and bedside manner.

Thyroidologists

Some doctors—not many—refer to themselves as thyroidologists. Officially, there really is no such thing as a thyroidologist, no official medically recognized group of professional "thyroidologists," or specialty known as thyroidology. Some endocrinologists use the term because their practice tends to focus heavily on thyroid patients versus the skew towards treating diabetes. In any case, a thyroidologist tends to be conventional, by-the-numbers type. Don't expect much in the way of complementary or alternative approaches here. It would be rare, for example, to find a thyroidologist that came out of an osteopathic medical school, or a holistic thyroidologist, for example.

Internists/General Practice/Primary Care Physicians

Internists and general practice, or family practice, docs are harder to group in terms of style or biases because they tend to come in all shapes and sizes. For many people, an internist or GP can do a fine job managing hypothyroidism, ordering regular TSH tests, and writing prescriptions for conventional thyroid drugs. If the doctor is an M.D. in a conventional medical practice, and particularly an HMO, it's pretty safe to assume to a large extent that the doctor will take a traditional approach, not unlike the endocrinologists, in managing thyroid problems. For those who do well under this conventional protocol, not much more is needed.

Rarer are the older family doctors, still versed in the use of Armour, who are open to prescribing it, knowing the success they've had with it for years. They're few and far between, but their patients are usually very loyal.

When you don't do well on the conventional approach, or when you want to understand more about the many side effects and symptoms of hypothyroidism, the fairly conventional focus of most internists and GPs may fall short of what you need.

Osteopathic Physicians/D.O.s

Currently, it's estimated that there are more than 30,000 American-educated and -licensed osteopathic physicians practicing in the United States. The majority of osteopaths physicians are in primary care—family medicine, pediatrics, internal medicine, and obstetrics-gynecology. Osteopaths have D.O. after their names, instead of M.D. Doctors of osteopathic medicine (D.O.s) are, for the most part, pretty hard to tell from an M.D. in many ways. D.O.s are "complete" physicians, fully trained and licensed to prescribe medication and to perform surgery. D.O.s and allopathic physicians (M.D.s) are the only two types of complete physicians. D.O.s are licensed in the same way as doctors, have to attend an osteopathic medical school, do internships and residencies. The main difference in is the philosophy of osteopathy versus conventional medicine. Osteopaths typically address people holistically, and instead of treating each symptom separately, look for the overall cause, and attempt to treat the whole person. Osteopathic physicians understand how all the body's systems are connected and related. Many osteopaths use physical manipulation of the musculoskeletal system.

Osteopaths have a reputation as good listeners and believe in helping patients develop attitudes and lifestyles that don't just fight illness, but help prevent it. In treating hypothyroidism, some osteopaths are conventional TSH/levothyroxine followers, but they're more likely to work with nontraditional prescription thyroid medicines, such as natural thyroid or the T3-related therapies. You'll also find them more open to herbs, vitamins, supplements, and other complementary therapies to help treat the underlying immune system or persistent symptoms.

Holistic Doctors

Holistic doctors focus on the whole person and how he or she interacts with the environment, rather than illness, disease, or specific body parts. A small number of M.D.s, and a larger percentage

of D.O.s, practice holistic medicine, following some general princi-
ples. They believe in prevention of disease when possible, and in
dealing with the underlying cause of a problem versus just treating
symptoms. They want to understand the patient as much as the
disease or illness, and diagnose patients as individuals, rather than
as "members of a disease category." They encourage patient auton-
omy—a doctor-patient relationship that considers the patient's
needs as much as the doctor's—and the healing power of love,
hope, humor, and other positive forces.

When it comes to hypothyroidism, holistic doctors are the most
likely to work with nontraditional prescription thyroid medicines,
such as natural thyroid or the T3-related therapies. They are also
more likely to be able to treat you using herbs, vitamins, supplements for your health related to the thyroid and immune system.

EVALUATING POTENTIAL DOCTORS

Most people will invest time in finding and evaluating a good me-
chanic, accountant, or babysitter. You need to take the same approach to finding a doctor. A medical diploma on the wall doesn't
guarantee that your doctor will be knowledgeable, have a positive
manner, or work effectively with you. It's up to you to find the
right doctor, within the constraints of your health plan, finances,
or geography.

Before you set out to choose a doctor, consider your main
priorities and selection criteria.

Cost/Coverage

For some people, going outside the HMO or insurance plan is
simply not a financial option. It's helpful to make this decision up
front, so you can narrow your search accordingly. If you are limited
to selecting doctors from a pre-approved list provided by your
HMO or health plan, you may want to start by asking your HMO
plan or insurance company if they offer any help in choosing from
their lists, or if they have further information on available doctors.
Otherwise, many of the other resources we'll discuss here can be

used to help "qualify" the doctors you do have available via your HMO or insurance plan.

Experience

How many years of experience you want depends on your preferences. Younger doctors may be more open to alternative medicine, for example, whereas older doctors might be more set in their ways, but more seasoned, experienced, with a better bedside manner.

Credentials

In some cases, you may want a doctor who graduated from a top conventional or osteopathic medical school. This isn't always an indicator of a good doctor, but the top echelon medical schools usually manage to weed out some of the worst students.

Certification

Being "board-certified" means a doctor has had several additional years of training in a particular specialty and passed a competency exam. Again, this doesn't guarantee that the doctor will be a success for you, but you're getting assurance of extra education in the particular specialty. When it comes to hypothyroidism, the main certification you might be looking for is "endocrinology."

Other Factors

Some other important factors include:

• *Record*—Some people want to make sure there are no disciplinary actions filed against a doctor, and there are ways to evaluate this.

• *Cutting Edge*—Some people want a doctor who is innovative and on the cutting edge, who reads all the journals and health reports, and keeps up with developments.

• *Style*—Some people prefer a respectful business style, others would rather have a warm, friendly doctor.

- *Conventional or Alternative Focus*—Some people balk at having a doctor who suggests acupuncture or herbal remedies, and others, conversely, wouldn't want a doctor who wasn't open to alternative therapies.

- *Gender*—Some people prefer to have a male or female doctor.

- *Flexibility*—Some people want a doctor who has evening or weekend hours, or who can see patients on short notice, or who will consult by phone.

- *Success*—Most people want a doctor who has successfully treated other patients with the same condition. This is usually information you can get only from other patients or perhaps from another doctor.

- *Recommendations*—You might want to talk to other patients who are satisfied customers. If a doctor is not willing to provide patient references, look somewhere else.

- *Referrals or Peer Recommendations*—You might want a doctor who has been recommended by other doctors. There are a variety of sources of this information that you can access.

I prefer a doctor who has a warm, participatory style, and is open to alternative and complementary therapies. You will have your own criteria. When looking for a doctor, Kathy, a thyroid cancer survivor, has a different focus, and looks for a doctor who is particularly up-to-date:

> Now that so much information is accessible via the Internet and on-line support groups, I want a doctor who is up-to-date on issues, research, treatment, etc. I don't like feeling I know more than the doctor does about my condition, the prescribed medication, and the options for testing and treatment. I also want my doctor to be receptive to my research. I don't like the attitude some doctors have that you can't possibly understand the topic at hand without a medical degree. I have B.S. and M.S. degrees, and while they're not in medi-

cine, I do understand scientific concepts and the scientific method of testing hypotheses. I'm also capable of reading an FDA report without having it interpreted by a pharmaceutical sales representative.

The Resources appendix has a number of helpful organizations, referral services, and Web sites that can help you find potential doctors.

SCREENING POTENTIAL DOCTORS TO CHOOSE THE RIGHT ONE

Once you've narrowed your selections and have a shortlist of possible doctors, it's time to have a brief screening interview by phone, during which you might want to ask the following sorts of questions:

- Are you accepting new patients and, if so, is a referral required?
- Are you an individual or group practice? If I have an appointment with you, is there a possibility I may be seen by another doctor without advance notice?
- Who covers for you when you're unavailable?
- On average, how long does a patient have to wait for an appointment? (How long in advance must I make an appointment?)
- Do you charge for missed appointments?
- Do you accept patient phone calls? Do you restrict them to any particular time of day? How soon do you typically return calls? Do you have your nurses return calls on your behalf?
- Is advice given over the phone?
- Do you accept patient emails?
- Do you accept patient faxes?
- What are your customary fees?
- Do you accept my health insurance coverage?
- Is full payment (or deductibles, co-payments) required at the time of the appointment?
- Do you take the time to explain treatment options, answer questions, and generally involve patients in their own treatment?
- Are lab work and x-rays performed in the office? Do you send blood samples out for TSH tests or do you perform them in house?

- What hours are you available?
- Do you refer patients to alternative treatments?
- Can you provide several patient references?

If a doctor's office isn't interested in at least providing you with some of this information in advance, or insists that you come in for a paid appointment to "interview" the doctor, then unless it's a doctor that you are very eager to see for many other reasons, I'd suggest moving on. Doctors who don't recognize that patients are clients to whom they provide a service often aren't productive in the long run.

There are other questions that unfortunately can't be answered until you are a patient. You may be able to get some ideas from other patients, but it's more likely you'll need to assess the doctor firsthand. Keep your ears and eyes open when talking to other patients, or when talking on the phone to the doctor's office, or during the initial visit for the following:

- Does your doctor patiently explain reasons for all tests and treatments?
- Does your doctor offer you any options?
- Does your doctor seem interested in educating you or just in giving orders to be followed?
- Does your doctor encourage you to participate in decisions about your health care?
- Does your doctor believe in alternative or complementary therapies?
- Does your doctor take time to learn about you, your background, your lifestyle, and how you truly feel?
- Does your doctor really listen?
- Does your doctor answer your questions satisfactorily?
- Does your doctor's receptionists, nurses, and other staff treat you and other patients politely and respectfully?
- Does your doctor and his or her staff let you dress and undress in private?
- Does your doctor or his or her staff gossip or share private information about other patients?

- Does your doctor admit or indicate that he or she just "isn't comfortable" with assertive or informed patients?
- Does your doctor take an authoritarian or dictatorial approach to the doctor-patient relationship?
- Does your doctor become irritated, act impatient, or ignore you when you ask for further explanation of your diagnosis, procedures to be performed, or drugs prescribed?
- Does your doctor return phone calls within a reasonable amount of time or tell you that he or she has left messages or tried to call when it's evident he or she hasn't?
- Does your doctor keep you waiting and usually run late for your appointments?
- When you mention some health finding you heard about on the evening news, does your doctor seem to be aware of it?
- Will your doctor read anything you provide to him or her as far as background information?
- Does your doctor categorically dismiss the "Internet" as a source of medical information?

Once you've settled on a doctor, your work is not done. Now you have to manage the relationship, ensuring that you are getting the best possible care.

Communicating Effectively with Your Doctor

David Elfstrom, author of an award-winning article, "How to Talk to Doctors," has several important tips on how to diplomatically and effectively communicate with your doctor. In my opinion, these are absolute necessities for all patients:

- Keep a medical diary of all significant health-related events.
- Educate yourself: Seek out new treatments. Know everything about the medications you are taking.
- Understand terminology using your medical dictionary.
- Write down a concise list of items to discuss before each appointment. Bring two copies.
- Don't bring any other photocopies, Internet printouts, or newspaper clippings to the meeting. Instead, fax them a few days

ahead with a polite note saying that you'd like to discuss them during your appointment.

- Be assertive rather than aggressive or passive.
- Be educated about your illness and symptoms, but leave the final diagnosing to your doctor.

Keeping Track of Your Medical/Health Information

Keeping a health diary between appointments can help you get the most out of appointments, and keep your health information organized. You can do this in a notebook, on the computer, or in folders. The form doesn't matter. The main concern is keeping track of appointments, copies of test results, and other pertinent information.

- *Doctor information:* Include the name, address, phone, fax, and email address for every doctor you see, even periodically. Keep track of receptionists' names. And also store directions to offices you don't visit frequently.

- *Pharmacy information:* Include the prescription numbers and number of refills available for all current prescriptions, plus phone numbers for your pharmacy or pharmacies.

- *Lab/treatment facility information:* Include the name, address, and phone number of any labs or treatment facilities (radiology labs, testing locations, and physical therapists.)

The diary should also keep track of your key health events, including illnesses, surgeries, and other pertinent information. A detailed health diary would include:

- dates of visits to the doctor
- dates when you've received any injections, vaccinations, or special treatments
- dates and locations of diagnostic procedures (TSH tests, x-rays, MRI, bone scan)
- dates starting and stopping a medication, and dosage levels

- blood test results—ask for a photocopy for your folder
- major emotional and physical stresses
- specific and unusual health symptoms—such as "today I felt cold and had a rapid pulse of 98," or "today, I was so tired I went to bed two hours early"

Paul, a registered nurse with hypothyroidism, has some excellent additional recommendations on what the health diary should include:

> The personal health diary should include date, time, duration (length of time), and quality (subjective description) of various symptoms, such as pain, palpitations, fever, hot flashes, sweats, and fatigue. Note the precipitating factors that cause the symptoms. Note what makes the symptoms better. Also note your daily diet, activity, sleep, and stresses (arguments, other health problems, financial concerns, marital stress). Having such a diary helped me with my Social Security disability claim, as well as helping my physicians help me with my illnesses.

As Paul mentioned, documenting your illnesses, bodily changes, persistent and unusual symptoms, and other health concerns makes it easier to effectively manage your health.

ENSURING SUCCESSFUL DOCTOR VISITS

A productive doctor's appointment is one during which you have a chance to cover your key concerns with the doctor. In many doctor's offices, time is at a premium, so a successful appointment requires advance preparation. Some ways to ensure your visit is as successful as possible include:

- Make up an agenda for your doctor's visit and bring two copies, one to share with the doctor. Be sure to include on your agenda all key questions, concerns, or unusual health symptoms. Writing down "difficult" questions sometimes makes it easier to ask them, and keeping track of key issues helps you remember all the things you want to cover with your doctor.

- Get in business mode. Act as if your appointment is a business meeting. You're the client, the doctor is the "contractor," so to speak. Doctors treat patients more respectfully when the patients dress professionally for the appointment, and when patients stay calm, relaxed and unemotional, and do not act apologetic or passive.

- Be sure to arrive on time. If you arrive in advance, don't spend time reading old magazines, spend the time reviewing your agenda and mentally preparing for your appointment.

- Take notes. It's hard to remember what the doctor says after an appointment, so jot down notes, names of things, instructions and other information, so you have a reference.

- Bring a friend. This can help you feel more relaxed with the doctor. If you doctor gives you a hard time about having a friend with you, this is a red flag. You're the patient, you're paying the bill, and you should be able to decide who you'd like in the examining room with you. Choose a friend who is able to speak up, but also diplomatic. Friends who are health professionals—or even doctors themselves—can be of particular help. Be sure your friend knows the agenda for the appointment, so he or she can remind you of points to cover, and can help remember details of what your doctor said or agreed to do.

❁   ❁   ❁

I hope that you are one of the people with an astute doctor who recognized signs of hypothyroidism right away, ordered the appropriate tests, interpreted them rationally, and started you quickly on the road to wellness. If that is not your experience, it may seem unfair that you need to learn about and understand the various ways of thyroid testing and diagnosis, manage your own health care situation, and even find a different doctor or perhaps pay out of pocket for thyroid testing. But please remember that being your own advocate may be the only way to get the proper diagnosis and care that will put you back on the path to living well.

CHAPTER 7

Complementary and Alternative Therapies for Hypothyroidism

Doctors don't know everything really. They understand matter, not spirit. And you and I live in spirit.
WILLIAM SAROYAN

"Researchers find garlic lowers cholesterol." "Studies show acupuncture can relieve pain." "New findings indicate prayer speeds healing." Today's health headlines make it clear that alternative medicine is no longer a New Age "fad." Alternative, or what is sometimes called complementary medicine, is an accepted part of today's mainstream health consciousness. The *Journal of the American Medical Association*, bastion of conventional medicine, reported that in 1997, Americans made more visits to alternative practitioners than to primary care doctors, and that in that same year, 40 percent of Americans used some form of alternative medicine, an almost 50 percent increase since 1990. The same journal devoted an entire issue in 1998 to alternative medicine research studies.

While many of us from conventionally oriented cultures find alternative medicine new, fresh and exciting compared to the norm, it's old news in other cultures. Holistic medical systems, herbal treatments, and mind-body medicine have been mainstays for thousands of years. In fact, only in the West does the term "alternative medicine" really mean anything. In countries like India or China, you don't usually have an either/or choice of alternatives. Day-to-day medicine in many countries simply blends Western-style medicine with what we could call alternative approaches.

Many of these cultures have discovered what Western society will realize in the twenty-first century: that the best medicine is a combination of all worlds, using effective alternative techniques *in conjunction with* conventional medicine.

This chapter is by no means a comprehensive overview of the many complementary and alternative ways to help support thyroid function, relieve symptoms, or in some cases even heal thyroid disease. That's an entire book in itself. What I present here comes from the experiences of many people with hypothyroidism, my own experiences, conversations with leading doctors and alternative practitioners, and research into alternative medicine and its impact on various illnesses, particularly when it relates to hypothyroidism. If a particular therapy or modality is not mentioned here, it does not mean that it doesn't work. It simply means I haven't found any research, heard from people who have tried it, tried it myself, or seen it recommended by respected practitioners . . . yet! But I continue to explore every interesting possibility and I will continue to report on any new alternative medicine developments in my newsletter and my Web sites.

Please note: For each therapy or form of alternative medicine covered in this chapter, the Resources appendix includes sources of additional information.

DO YOU NEED ALTERNATIVE MEDICINE?

If you're reading this book, it's probably because you are one of the millions of people who have found that the "take this levothyroxine pill, see me in a year" approach to managing hypothyroidism is not working for you. It's always essential to get at the root issue, which means you need to be sure that you're on the *right* thyroid hormone replacement (for you . . . not for your doctor or the pharmaceutical companies) and at the right TSH level for you. But if you're truly stuck in a medical system that allows no options in terms of the thyroid hormone replacement, or you've explored all the traditional medical avenues and still aren't living well, then it might be time to look at complementary and alternative medicine to help deal with the issue of overall health or specific symptoms.

If you're not already a devotee of alternative medicine, before you launch in, there are some questions you should probably ask yourself:

- Why do I want to try alternative medicine?
- What are my expectations?
- Have I considered some available options and decided on one approach (i.e., massage or yoga) or will I pursue more general treatment via a particular medical system, i.e., Traditional Chinese Medicine, or leave it up to a practitioner like a holistic M.D. or naturopath to recommend alternative therapies?
- Do I understand the type of alternative medicine I'll be using?
- Do I have a complete understanding of the costs, including herbs, treatments, books, tapes, classes, or other recommended materials and preparations that might be part of the recommended therapy?
- How much time and money am I willing to spend before I feel as if the alternative therapy has worked?
- Have I told my primary care physician? (If not, it's usually a good idea.)

The final and key question you need to ask yourself is if you are ready to truly commit to an alternative therapy. Some of them are not easy to follow. You may be asked to completely change your diet and give up meat, or sugar, or bread products, for example. Or you'll need to take dozens of capsules and herbal preparations a day. You need commitment and patience. Alternative therapies rarely offer a quick fix. It may take longer to heal and normalize things using alternative therapies, so you have to be prepared for this possibility.

If you are determined to forge ahead, start by finding an alternative practitioner recommended by your physician, trusted health advisors, or other patients. If there are licensing or certifications associated with the particular alternative therapy, it's always wise to select a practitioner who has the appropriate credentials. If you're not familiar with the form of alternative medicine or the practitioner, you might want to have an initial meeting, during which you can find out more, including:

- the practitioner's experience and background
- how familiar the practitioner is with your health problem, success rates, typical approaches, and even patient referrals
- time frames for treatment

- costs
- what is involved in the treatment

Just as it was suggested in chapter 6 that you take a rigorous approach to selecting a doctor, that same approach should be used in choosing alternative practitioners.

IS THERE A NATURAL "TREATMENT" FOR HYPOTHYROIDISM?

Many people want to know if there's a natural or alternative treatment for hypothyroidism that doesn't require a doctor's treatment or a prescription. At present, there is no plant or herbal replacement for thyroid hormone. Some people with a mild depression decide to get some St. John's Wort instead of seeing a doctor and going on Prozac. It's not like that with hypothyroidism. There is no natural or over-the-counter herb or supplement that acts like thyroid hormone and can be taken instead of thyroid hormone. There are things that "help" the thyroid or the immune system function better, and in some cases, practitioners claim herbs, supplements, or other treatments can restore an underfunctioning thyroid to normal. But that is different from a "natural" thyroid hormone replacement.

When people refer to "natural" thyroid hormone, they are talking about Armour Thyroid, Westhroid, or Naturethroid, prescription thyroid hormone replacement drugs made from the desiccated thyroid glands of pigs. "Natural thyroid" does not refer to over-the-counter or multilevel-marketing "glandular" supplements, made with raw thyroid and other endocrine glands of cattle and pigs. These glandular products are not providing consistent amounts of thyroid hormone and could, in fact, pose a slight danger of "Mad Cow Disease," or other sorts of problems. Some people attempt to diagnose and treat themselves by taking these glandular supplements, but this can be risky. You should at least establish with a health practitioner that you do have a thyroid problem, then you can investigate alternative approaches. Glandulars should not be taken unless you are under the guidance of a knowledgeable health professional who strongly recommends them and can vouch for a particular brand.

CHINESE MEDICINE/ACUPUNCTURE

Chinese Medicine (CM) originated from Taoism about 4,000 years ago. CM is a treatment designed to balance the health of an individual and his or her surroundings. Central to that balance is *qi* (pronounced "chee"), which translates as "vital energy" or "life force." Qi flows through the body via pathways known as meridians and is exchanged with the body's surroundings. A body is in optimal health when qi is free and balanced. In addition to qi, CM relies on the concept of yin and yang, the interdependent opposites, representing different organs and health aspects. CM diagnostic techniques include observation, listening, questioning, and palpation, including feeling special pulse qualities and sensitivity of body parts. CM treatments include diet, exercises such as T'ai Chi and the Qi Gong breathing, herbal preparations, acupuncture, acupressure massage, physical therapy, and moxibustion. Moxibustion is the use of heat at specific energy points on the body—applied either directly or to the acupuncture needles—as a way to add energy.

In the U.S., acupuncture is now an established practice, both as part of CM and even more so on its own. Americans make an estimated nine to twelve million visits to acupuncturists annually, and some 3,000 conventionally trained U.S. physicians also practice acupuncture.

Acupuncture requires inserting very thin, fine needles at different key energy points to regulate or correct the flow of qi and restore health. Acupuncture treatment taps into points along meridians, each having different therapeutic functions within the body. Most of the time, patients don't feel the acupuncture needles at all; occasionally, the worst they might feel is a slight pinch for a second. As a regular recipient of acupuncture treatment, and someone who really doesn't like shots, I can tell you that despite how it looks, when done properly acupuncture does not hurt. It's also safe. Most practitioners use disposable needles, and it's a good idea to ask your acupuncturist to use them.

Acupuncture has been well studied and proven to be effective for a variety of problems. In 1997, the National Institute of Health Consensus Development Conference on Acupuncture, found that pain from musculoskeletal conditions and nausea were successfully treated with acupuncture. In late 1998, a University of Arizona study also found acupuncture an aid in treatment for depression.

There are many verified studies conducted in Asia that show successful application of CM for immunologically based diseases, including thyroid problems. Specifically regarding hypothyroidism, a study in the *Journal of Chinese Medicine* found that use of moxibustion along with Chinese medicinal powder at specific energy points led to recovery of thyroid function in some patients with Hashimoto's thyroiditis. Another study showed that treatment with Shen Lu Tablets could address the underling yin deficiencies that are at the root of some hypothyroidism, actually lowering TSH levels and reducing symptoms. Various Chinese medical herbal tonics have also been studied and found to have an effect on TSH levels and hypothyroid symptoms. Acupuncture can also be very effective in treating the deficiency of deep energy—yin—that is so common in hypothyroidism, and in some of the symptomatic pain that can accompany hypothyroidism or related fibromyalgia.

I have personally found that only regular weekly acupuncture sessions help me through episodes of severe fatigue and total exhaustion. Whenever I start suffering from unusually low energy, I go in for a few weekly sessions, and things get back to normal and my energy becomes more balanced.

Kate Lemmerman, M.D., makes acupuncture a key part of her medical practice. She finds that 60 to 70 percent of her patients with fatigue from hypothyroidism and other causes experience benefit from acupuncture treatments. How acupuncture adds energy, however, is not easy to explain:

> Asians may say that we miss the forest for the trees when we try to explain how acupuncture works in terms of endorphins, cortisol, and serotonin. Suffice it to say that by balancing the qi, roughly translated as energy, in someone's system, we allow improved functioning and healing. And that by using certain "tonifying" techniques, such as heating the needles, we can actually add energy. . . .

When choosing an acupuncturist, be sure to see someone who is licensed and certified, whether a doctor or not. For physicians, top certification is from the American Academy of Medical Acupuncture (AAMA). Acupuncturists, who are not doctors, can receive credentials known as a Diplomate in Acupuncture (Dipl.Ac.). They may be called Licensed Acupuncturist (L.Ac. or Lic.Ac.), Registered Acupuncturist (R.Ac.), Certified Acupuncturist (C.A), Acupuncturist, Doctor of Oriental Medicine (DOM), or Doctor of Acupuncture (D.Ac.) Each state has its own specific requirements for practice of acupuncture. Either see a licensed acupuncturist or one who is nationally certified from an organization like the National Certification Commission for Acupuncture and Oriental Medicine (NCCAOM).

AYURVEDA

Ayurveda (pronounced AH-yuhr-vey-duh) has been the traditional medicine of India for more than 5,000 years and is probably the oldest medical system in existence. Ayurveda is a Sanskrit word that means "science of life" or "life knowledge" and is based on the premise that the body naturally seeks harmony and balance. In Ayurveda, disease represents emotional imbalance, toxins in the body, and most particularly, imbalances in what are known as *doshas*. Doshas are different regulatory systems—vata (movement), pitta (heat, metabolism, and energy), and kapha (physical structure and fluid balance) that govern different aspects of health. According to Ayurveda, proper balancing of the doshas is accomplished through food and diet, herbs, meditation and breathing, massage, and even yoga poses to ensure that energy is flowing. In this way, the concept of balance and energy makes it similar to Chinese medicine.

Some naturopaths and homeopaths offer aspects of Ayurvedic treatment, or incorporate ayurvedic herbal preparations as part of their treatments. There are also purely Ayurvedic practitioners. Typically, Ayurvedic practitioners make a diagnosis by asking detailed questions to assess your dominant dosha, and take ayurvedic pulses.

As far as applicability to hypothyroidism, when something affects as many aspects of health as hypothyroidism does, therapies that focus on balancing of all the systems can be particularly useful, and Ayurveda is no exception. Ayurveda has much to offer, and to truly benefit from Ayurveda, it's worthwhile to consult a trained practitioner or Ayurvedic doctor for an evaluation and recommendations.

Ayurvedic therapy is considered particularly effective for disease brought on or exacerbated by stress, for energy and improved breathing and respiration, and for weight loss. These strengths apply to some of the most common hypothyroidism-related symptoms.

Z-guggulsterone, a component derived from the plant commiphora mukul, has been used as an important antiinflammatory, antiobesity, and cholesterol-lowering agent in a popular Ayurvedic medicine known as "guggul." Guggul is considered particularly important for prevention of a sluggish metabolism, and studies have shown that Z-guggulsterone has the ability to increase the thyroid's ability take up the enzymes it needs for effective hormone conversion. It also increases the oxygen uptake in muscles. Some Ayurvedic practitioners have reported tremendous success with use of guggul products.

Constipation is often a problem with hypothyroidism. One of the most basic and classic Ayurvedic herbal remedies is known as "triphala," and many thyroid patients report that daily use of triphala can have a remarkable impact on digestion and constipation problems. Various triphala preparations are available at many natural health and vitamin stores.

Ayurvedic practitioners are not officially licensed, but you should ask where and how long a practitioner was trained, how long he or she's been practicing Ayurveda, and how much of his or her practice is purely Ayurveda.

HERBAL MEDICINE

When you pick up a bottle of echinacea off the supermarket shelf or drink a ginger ale to settle your stomach, you're actually practicing a form of herbal medicine. Going back to the most ancient times, there has been a well-developed understanding of the power of plants and plant products as medicine. Many of today's drugs are actually derived from herbal sources or are synthetic versions of naturally occurring herbs. According to the World Health Organization (WHO) about four billion people, or 80 percent of the world's population, use some form of herbal medicine.

While always a mainstay in the East, herbal medicine is becoming popular again in the West, with a variety of treatments taken as teas, as capsules or tablets, extracts or tinctures, and essential oils for topical use. In the United States, herbal medicine practitioners may be physicians, osteopaths, naturopaths, nutritionists, or even more traditional herbalists. Be very wary, however, of the new crop of so-called herbalists who have popped up around the massive multilevel-marketing vitamin business. Armies of salespeople are hawking all sorts of herbs and supplements, but their main credential is their membership in some sort of multilevel network marketing company, and their desire to sell you a whole boatload of products you probably don't need.

Many medical studies in the U.S., Europe, and Asia have found that legitimate herbal products can have an impact on health conditions, ranging from liver repair, to enhancing the immune system to reducing swelling to increasing energy or aiding in weight loss.

Herbal and aromatherapy expert Mindy Green of the Herbal Research Foundation has some interesting recommendations about the use of herbs for energy, stimulation, or adrenal support:

> We live in a society that runs on stimulation—whether it's coffee, or violence on television—things that make us live on that edge. So while there are some excellent herbs and essential oils for adrenal support, people need to take care not to try these products along with other stimulants. When you're trying to tone your adrenals, you don't want to drink caffeine, or watch horror movies or violent news stories, for example. Instead of the simulating effect of aerobics, do something more calming, like yoga or T'ai Chi. It's almost as if you need to train your body to run more on internal energy than outside energy and stimulation.

The way Mindy described it was that taking excessive stimulants when your endocrine or adrenal systems are depleted is "like kicking a dead horse."

From an herbal standpoint, Mindy recommends Siberian ginseng, as opposed to regular ginseng, and astragalus, which is also good for immune support, as key tonics for the adrenal and endocrine systems.

In her book *Herbal Defense,* author and herbalist Robyn Landis discusses the benefits of Siberian ginseng and astragalus, and also recommends several other herbs for thyroid support:

- fo-ti root (Ho Shou Wu) a Chinese herb that's broader and slower in action than—but similar to—ginseng
- saw palmetto berry, as a thyroid tonic
- the Ayurvedic remedy triphala, as a long-term, glandular tonic
- black cohosh root, as a long-term, glandular tonic

Stress reduction and relaxation can both help the overall immune system. The Herb Research Foundation's Mindy Green recommends the tea forms of several herbs, including chamomile, and melissa, which is also known as lemon balm, as relaxing herbal tonics. Mindy suggests that an easy way for a beginner to try relaxing tea is to get something like Sleepytime Tea, by Celestial Seasonings.

I asked her what, as a person with hypothyroidism, I should reach for when I'm just completely out of steam and am ready for a giant double espresso in order to make it through the day. Mindy, said, unquestionably, maté tea.

Maté, pronounced, "mah-TAY," is an herbal tea native to South America. Maté is considered far more nutritious than black tea or coffee, and though it also has some caffeine, it's effects are energizing. It doesn't make people jittery. On the scale of bad to good, coffee should be your last choice, followed by black tea, then green tea. Maté is the best option.

The Issue of Kelp and Iodine

It seems that for every alternative practitioner you find who recommends that people take iodine or kelp for their thyroid, there's one who disagrees. Traditionally, some herbalists and alternative practitioners have recommended iodine-containing herbs or supplements, such as bladderwrack and bugleweed, in order to help thyroid function. They argue that more iodine than is typically taken in by the regular diet is needed for proper thyroid function. Categorically, many of them state that if the thyroid isn't functioning properly, it needs iodine in some form.

A study reported in the *Journal of Clinical Endocrinology and Metabolism* in late 1998 indicated that over the past twenty years, the percentage of Americans with low intake of iodine has more than quadrupled. Currently about 12 percent of the U.S. population is iodine deficient, up from less than 3 percent in the early 1970s. So, for some people, iodine deficiency may be a factor in their thyroid problem.

At the same time, some alternative and conventional practitioners have found that iodine or iodine-containing herbal products make people with an autoimmune thyroid problem feel far worse, causing a "crash" of energy. Under the care of a homeopathic doctor, I, too, tried iodine supplements, and it made me feel *terrible* for two weeks, so I discontinued them. I tried again on my own with a metabolism/thyroid support supplement that contained iodine. Again, within a day or two, I was *exhausted* and after a week, barely functional. A third time, again it had a terrible effect. Personally, I've given up trying iodine. I've had many similar reports from others. While my correspondence is not an accurate poll or research into iodine, I've had only a handful of people who say they've had success with iodine. Far more common are the reports that it has caused major crashes, and days of complete fatigue and exhaustion.

It's been suggested that if iodine products are taken in conjunction with other supplements—such as selenium—the iodine does help thyroid function, and doesn't cause a negative crash. These subjects could benefit from further research.

If you would like to find an herbalist, keep in mind that a fair number of naturopaths and holistic doctors are also herbal medicine practitioners, and can both diagnose and recommend treatments. Without a medical license, an herbalist is technically not permitted to make a diagnosis. There's no official licensing for herbalists, so be sure you've checked out your herbalist and are satisfied that you are selecting someone qualified to treat you. Generally, you can expect some level of professionalism from any herbalist who is a member of the American Herbalists Guild, so ask about this affiliation.

NUTRITIONAL AND VITAMIN THERAPY

If you've taken a vitamin C capsule or drank a big glass of orange juice at the sign of cold, or eaten extra garlic to help your cholesterol level, then you are practicing nutritional and vitamin therapy.

Dietary and nutrition are basic aspects of many of the complementary and alternative medicine systems, such as Ayurveda or Traditional Chinese Medicine. In fact, many healing methods look at food as a medicine much like a pill from a pharmacy.

From a dietary standpoint, therapies can include macrobiotic diets, vegetarian or vegan diets, low-glycemic diets, or individualized dietary programs that add or take away certain foods or food groups. Nutritionally, vitamin, mineral, and enzyme supplements replace missing nutrients, or megavitamin therapies used to prevent or treat particular health problems.

There are so many possible combinations of nutritional therapies, and so many different diets, vitamins, minerals, and supplements one could take, that it's not possible to cover them here. But we know that diet and supplements can have a direct impact on blood pressure, obesity, heart disease, allergies, fatigue and exhaustion, chronic yeast infections, sleep problems, skin disruptions, osteoporosis, and premenstrual syndrome, among many health concerns.

If you take your multivitamin every day, you may think you're getting what you need for optimal health. Many nutritional experts, however, feel that "minimum daily requirements" are not sufficient to prevent chronic diseases, or help heal you when your health is compromised by an ongoing battle with hypothyroidism. Some experts believe that some forms of hypothyroidism actually reflect underlying nutritional deficiencies that, when corrected, may restore thyroid function.

As far as nutritional and vitamin therapies for hypothyroidism, there's no way that I can sit down and tell you what particular mix of vitamins, foods, nutritional supplements, herbs, or other natural remedies will be right to address your hypothyroidism, or related unresolved symptoms. You can try hit-or-miss self-medication, as many people do. But you'll save yourself time and money, and get far closer to the right combinations, if you start out with a visit to a respected and recommended nutritionist with expertise in working with thyroid problems.

Nutritional Issues for Hypothyroidism

A nutritionist I've consulted, Dana Godbout Laake, is a nationally known expert on working with vitamins, minerals, and supplements. She addresses the nutritional deficiencies that cause—or accompany—diseases such as hypothyroidism, fibromyalgia, chronic fatigue, and rheumatoid arthritis. Dana feels that vitamin deficiencies need to be addressed and healed before thyroid problems can often be truly resolved. When there are underlying nutritional or digestion problems, the thyroid hormone isn't properly absorbed, making it inaccessible to the body. In essence, no matter what thyroid drug you're taking or how much of it you take, if your body can't absorb it properly to start, then achieving thyroid balance is more difficult.

In *Prescription for Nutritional Healing*, authors Dr. James Balch and nutritionist Phyllis Balch recommend L-tyrosine. L-tyrosine is a known precursor to thyroid hormone, and apparently, low levels can be associated with hypothyroidism. A few of the other recommendations made by the Balches are:

- B complex, including B_2 and extra B_{12}
- Brewer's Yeast, to provide B vitamins and extra nutrients. (Note, you need to watch taking this if you have a tendency to yeast/candidiasis.)
- Essential fatty acids, for thyroid function
- Vitamin C, approximately 2,000 mg a day. Note that this is a fair amount. They recommend taking no more than this, as megadoses can affect the production of thyroid hormone.
- Vitamin E, for immune and thyroid function
- Zinc, for immune and thyroid function

In an article titled "Energizing Chronic Fatigue" that appeared in *Alternative Medicine* magazine, noted alternative practitioner Rafael Kellman, M.D. has identified that many people with chronic fatigue have a variety of vitamin deficiencies. He notes the main ones he finds are deficiencies of vitamin C and the B-complex vitamins. In the article, it indicates that he frequently recommends:

- L-tyrosine, the precursor to the T4 thyroid hormone
- Up to 3000 mg of vitamin C daily
- Extensive vitamin B complex supplementation
- Magnesium supplements
- The Chinese herb astragalus, as a tonic for strengthening the immune system, making it better able to fight disease and infection.

According to Ted Huston, a Ph.D. chemist with thyroid disease himself who studies thyroid-related vitamin and nutritional deficiencies and treatments as an avocation, vitamins B_1 and B_2 are essential to overall health with hypothyroidism.

> Two critical vitamins, B_1 and B_2, are linked forever with the energy metabolism that our thyroids are trying to regulate. Vitamin B_1 is essential to carbohydrate metabolism and is absolutely required during fasting to maintain basal metabolism. B_2 is involved in the metabolism of thyroid hormones; specifically, it catalyzes the deiodination of thyroxine (T4) to liothyronine (T3).

Another vitamin issue to consider is getting enough, but not too much, selenium. Research has shown that selenium is an important mineral for thyroid function. In recent research, scientists have determined that the conversion of T4 to T3 is also controlled by selenium. Selenium activates an enzyme responsible for controlling thyroid function by the conversion of T4 to T3. T4 is converted to T3 by something called "hepatic type I iodothyronine deiodinase," a selenoprotein that is sensitive to selenium deficiency.

A 1997 study also suggests that high intake of iodine when selenium is deficient may permit thyroid damage. An intake of selenium appeared to offset the effect of high iodine intake on thyroid function. Stress and injury appear to make the body particularly thyroid-responsive and selenium-deficient. After severe injury, T4 deiodination is decreased, leading to low T3 syndrome. A research study found that selenium levels are low after trauma, which correlates to low T3 levels, along with a decrease in the T4 to T3 conversion.

Finally, evening primrose oil (also known as EPO) is another nutritional supplement that is frequently mentioned. In his book,

Solved: The Riddle of Illness, Stephen Langer, M.D. points out that symptoms of essential fatty acid insufficiency are very similar to hypothyroidism, and recommends evening primrose oil—an excellent source of essential fatty acids—for people with hypothyroidism. Endocrinologist Kenneth Blanchard, M.D., recommends EPO for his patients with hair loss. When there's a sex pattern to hair loss— if a woman is losing hair in partly a male pattern—he believes the problem is excessive conversion of testosterone to dihydrotestosterone at the level of the hair follicle. Evening primrose oil is an inhibitor of that conversion.

As someone who has had a few periods of extensive hair loss since become hypothyroid, I can vouch for the fact that taking EPO was the only thing that calmed it down.

How to Take Vitamins and Supplements

Before running for the vitamin bottles, Ted, along with many nutritional experts, recommends starting with the dinner plate:

> Is your diet balanced? The answer is, of course, "who knows?" Consider whether you are eating enough of all the food groups. Many of the B vitamins have principal sources in meat/dairy products; are you a vegetarian and carefully accounting for this? Are you eliminating fat from your diet? This has consequences to the fat-soluble vitamins, A, D, E, and K. Also, you need to increase intake of B_1 if fat is less than about 40 percent of caloric intake. Eating is supposed to be fun. Don't try to replace it with a pill. We aren't the Jetsons.

Ted also has some excellent advice on how to ensure that you're getting the best quality vitamins:

> Look for the USP symbol or other national recognition label. It is sort of like the UL label on household appliances. It ensures a minimum level of quality and that there are indeed the levels of vitamins reported on the label. You are free to spend as much or little on them as you are comfortable with. I know there are many of you who are putting your health food store owner's children through college, and you are paying for their boats. Fine. It is your choice and your

bank account. The issue of natural versus synthetic is bound to come up. Choose your path as you wish. A rose hip by any other name would smell as sweet.

One piece of advice that is valuable for anyone taking vitamins is to take your vitamins with food. A very basic reason is that many people will become nauseous if they take vitamins on an empty stomach. Most vitamins require stomach acids and gastric juices to convert them into absorbable or useful forms.

If you choose to go to a professional nutritionist, major accreditations to look for include:

- R.D.—Registered Dietician: Granted by the Commission on Dietetic Registration to graduates of four-year colleges and universities with dietary programs accredited by the American Dietetic Association
- C.N.C.—Certified Nutritional Consultant: Issued by the American Association of Nutritional Consultants

NATUROPATHY

Naturopathy draws on aspects of Traditional Chinese Medicine, Ayurveda, and other medical systems for its focus. Naturopathic philosophy aims for a balance of physical, emotional, mental, and spiritual aspects, highlighting the body's innate ability to heal itself. Naturopathic doctors act like primary care providers for many complementary therapies and are often well connected to a network of alternative providers.

Naturopathy seeks to identify and treat root causes of illness or the disease process instead of symptoms. Naturopaths may recommend, or themselves practice, acupuncture, homeopathy, herbal medicine, dietary and nutritional medicine, manipulation or massage, and other techniques. It's estimated that there are more than 1,000 naturopathic doctors in practice in the United States.

Since naturopathic medicine draws on many different disciplines, there are certainly arguments to be made for its effectiveness. But since there's no specific "naturopathic" remedies or treatments, it really is up to the individual practitioner to achieve results.

Some patients have written to me to recommend Zafirah Ahmed, N.D., an Arizona-based naturopathic doctor. Dr. Ahmed, who has Graves' disease herself, uses special testing to assess whether a thyroid problem can be corrected with glandular supplements or whether it is an adrenal problem.

She also reports having success treating the following symptoms with corresponding supplements:

- hypoglycemia—chromium, vanadium, and gymna slyvestry
- hair loss—aromatherapy formulas for baldness.
- carpal tunnel syndrome—hand braces and aromatherapy formulas.

If you are looking for a naturopath, stick with someone who has an "N.D." and is a licensed Doctor of Naturopathic Medicine. The Council on Naturopathic Medical Education grants this designation after completion of a four-year program at one of the several accredited naturopathic colleges in the U.S.

MANUAL HEALING/BODYWORK

If you've ever had a massage and enjoyed the relaxed, warm feeling you have for many hours afterward, you've enjoyed the health benefits of manual healing and bodywork. This is a broad category that focuses on the use of touch to heal the body. Massage and manipulation are some of the oldest methods of health care. In bodywork, manual techniques, using hands, arms, elbows, and sometimes even feet, apply various types of pressure to affect the muscles, bones, joints, circulation, and other body systems.

There are so many different forms of massage and manual-healing that it's hard to list them all. Swedish massage, trigger point massage (myotherapy, neuromuscular massage therapy), Rolfing, Trager, Alexander technique, Feldenkrais, myofascial-release technique, and other realignment therapies concentrate on the soft tissue surrounding the bones. Practitioners of reflexology and acupressure stimulate points to clear energy pathways that appear to be blocked. And there are many kinds of energetic work, such as Reiki and Therapeutic Touch, in which the therapist is a conduit for healing energy that is directed to the patient through the therapist's hands, sometimes without actually touching the client.

Sandy Levy is an experienced bodywork expert who runs her own myotherapy practice. She has some thoughts about choosing the right therapy:

> Any type of bodywork can be useful. It's more important to find a good therapist with whom you are comfortable than a practitioner of a certain technique. To begin, ask yourself whether your body desires deep massage or a lighter touch . . . and follow your body's advice. Then ask around for referrals. If you want light massage, you will be looking for someone who specializes in Swedish massage and stress reduction, or one of the energy therapies like acupressure. If you crave deeper work, look for deep massage, or trigger point work, or, if you want to go all the way, Rolfing.

Sandy has found that more than one technique can sometimes be the best solution. In her practice, she provides light, relaxing massage, deep trigger point work, plus energetic therapies like Reiki and reflexology. And she's found that many of her clients also need movement/posture work, and she refers them to Alexander or Feldenkrais practitioners.

Before choosing one, talk with several therapists about their work so you can get a feel for whether you think you can work with them. The therapist should be willing to give you at least some telephone time, but you might want to pay for a brief office consult if you have many questions.

Bodywork can be quite helpful for unresolved hypothyroid symptoms, particularly if the therapist is familiar with the disease and is able to offer a combination of techniques. Medical studies have found various forms of massage and physical therapy to be effective in dealing with pain, depression, energy, insomnia, and inflammation. Some myofascial and myotherapy experts have had particular success working with the fibromyalgia and chronic fatigue symptoms that can also plague people with hypothyroidism.

Sandy has worked with many patients with hypothyroidism:

Massage—deep or light, depending on the person—is very helpful in relieving muscle aches and edema, but if the therapist can also stimulate the endocrine system via acupressure or reflexology or some other energetic method, the results will be much better.

There are different licensing and accreditation requirements for each type of bodywork. Many specialty areas—such as Rolfing and Feldenkrais—offer separate certification. Some states and areas license massage therapists. The main certification to look for, however, is N.C.T.M.B., which is granted by the National Certification Board for Therapeutic Massage and Bodywork, after completion of 500 hours of training and passage of an exam.

OSTEOPATHIC MANIPULATION

Osteopathic manipulation works with the musculoskeletal system as a way to treat illness, which in osteopathic theory, can result from imbalances and misalignment in the body's structure. As part of their broader family practice functions, many osteopathic physicians rely on this osteopathic manipulation as a form of treatment. Some M.D. practitioners have also been trained in osteopathic manipulation and can provide this sort of therapy.

There is clear research supporting the use of osteopathic manipulation and techniques for musculoskeletal and nonmusculoskeletal problems. Osteopathic manipulation is particularly useful for muscular and joint pain relief and for hypothyroidism-related problems, such as carpal tunnel syndrome or chronic sinusitis. Personally, I've found osteopathic manipulation to be most useful in dealing with various muscle trauma and joint pain, such as a case of whiplash I had after being rear-ended in my car. The manipulation allowed fewer painkillers and muscle relaxants, and sped up the healing process.

If you want to find an osteopath, you'll definitely need someone who has a D.O. degree from a four-year institution accredited by the American Association of Colleges of Osteopathic Medicine.

MIND-BODY THERAPY

Mind-body therapy is a broad category that looks at everything from prayer to yoga to counseling to dance to breathing. Basically, they are all practices or therapies that seek to establish a link between conscious thought and the body with the goal of affecting physiological processes.

Typically, mind-body therapies fall into two categories: physical therapies, such as dance, or mental therapies, such as biofeedback, or therapies that combine aspects of both, such as yoga, or T'ai Chi. Mind-body work also includes imagery, hypnosis, transcendental meditation, psychotherapy, prayer/spiritual healing, music therapy, art therapy, breathing exercises, humor therapy, and other forms of relaxation.

Sometimes the effectiveness of these therapies is written off as the "placebo" effect, but that overlooks its effectiveness. If we believe that unconscious thought—general stress, for example, or negative self-talk—can cause illness, why wouldn't we think that conscious, positive thought could help ward off illness or heal the body? Rather than simply serving as a placebo, there is also a strong medical basis for mind-body therapy. Recent studies in the field of psychoneuroimmunology show that the mind can communicate with the nervous, immune, and endocrine systems via cells called neurotransmitters. Various chemical and hormonal releases can then affect health and physical function as a result of conscious thought.

Research shows that mind-body techniques are particularly useful in the stress-reduction areas, helping to reduce blood pressure, pain, headaches, asthma, and other illnesses with a strong stress component. Mind-body techniques are also empowering, involving you in your own health care as an active participant.

There are so many types of mind-body therapy that we can just touch upon a few. You'll need to more fully research those therapies that are most appealing to you and where best to participate.

• *Psychotherapy or counseling*, by providing an outlet for stress and anxiety, can help to calm down your overall emotional state, allowing more energy for healing, more positive thoughts and actions, which in turn speeds recovery.

• *Support groups* also provide an outlet for anxiety and stress. They have the added benefit of, in many cases, providing education and information that gives you a feeling of greater control. Studies have even found that people with fatal illnesses live far longer when they are part of a support group.

• *Meditation techniques* are most common in Asia and are an integral part of Buddhism, Hinduism, yoga, and many Asian religions. They have gained popularity in other countries in the past thirty years. Regular meditation or *guided relaxation and imagery* have notable effects on blood pressure, anxiety, chronic pain, and can clinically reduce cortisol levels, a measure of the body's stress.

• *Biofeedback* is a treatment method that uses monitoring instruments to feed back to patients various physical information—such as pulse, body temperature, and other indicators of stress—which they normally don't monitor. By wearing the biofeedback monitor, they learn to adjust their thinking and other processes to control blood pressure, temperature, gastrointestinal functioning, and brain wave activity. Biofeedback is particularly effective at treating stress, sleep disorders, headaches, and high blood pressure.

• *Creative therapies—such as dance, music, or art*—use creative and physical activities to address health concerns. Creative therapies are particularly good for treating stress and blood pressure disorders.

• *Prayer and mental healing techniques* usually describe an altered state of consciousness due to a spiritual experience, or the "flow of energy" or healing via another person's hands. Studies have shown these techniques can be effective, again particularly when it comes to stress and energy-related problems.

YOGA

While yoga is a therapy that technically falls both into the "mind-body" category and is related to Ayurveda, I've covered it separately because I feel it is an important alternative therapy for people with hypothyroidism.

When most people think of yoga, they assume it means stretching or sitting in a cross-legged lotus position. Yoga is actually an ancient science that focuses on putting the whole body, mind, and intellect in harmony with the universe. This may sound like New Age babble, but, actually, yoga is quite practical, with physical exercises (known as asanas), breathing exercises (pranayama) and meditation techniques that help achieve that union and balance.

Some of the many health benefits of yoga have been conventionally tested and proven, and are even discussed in Western medical journals. For example, certain forms of yoga have been found to have a strong antidepressant effect. Yoga has also been found to improve lung function and breathing, and significantly reduce the amount of asthma medicines needed by asthmatic patients. Yoga is also considered an effective treatment for carpal tunnel syndrome. These are just a few of the many practical applications even mainstream medicine has found for yoga.

To find out more about yoga and its impact on thyroid disease and metabolism, I spoke with a well-respected yogi, Swami Rameshwarananda, who runs the Yoga in Daily Life Center in Alexandria, Virginia. Yoga in Daily Life is an internationally known comprehensive yoga system founded by Paramhans Swami Maheshwarananda and includes a set of recommendations of how to achieve balance of mind and spiritual harmony. I started yoga classes with Swami Rameshwarananda in mid-1998 and have been a fairly faithful practitioner ever since. In my neverending quest for wellness—on a variety of levels—I have to say that yoga has been one of the most satisfying, rewarding, and *effective* things I've done.

Yoga is not a quick fix solution for hypothyroidism, but it offers some overall health benefits, as well as some very specific benefits for metabolism and thyroid function. Yoga is about union of body, mind, and spirit. The word yoga means union, and in yoga, exercises, breath energy (prana), and meditation are all practiced in order to achieve that union and balance. In yoga, disease—such as hypothyroidism—represents a lack of unity somewhere in the "body." But to yogis, the body is not just physical. There are five distinct bodies, or planes that interact with each other:

- nourishment/physical body
- energy
- mind
- intellect
- causality, bliss

In yoga, a disease can represent a lack of harmony in the physical body or evidence of lack of harmony in the mind. Western medicine, on the contrary, typically focuses on the purely physical causes of illness. Swami Rameshwarananda greatly respects allopathic medicine but feels that much of it focuses on the body of nourishment:

> The focus is on eating, taking in nutrients, and how those nutrients are broken down to various chemicals. The other "bodies" are not considered much. The objective of yoga is balance of the whole system . . . harmony among *all* the bodies.

Yoga also looks at energy and life force in a unique way. In yoga, each of us has eight main chakras. While the direct translation of the word chakra is "wheel," it's more accurate to think of it as an energy vortex that concentrates energy in and out of our selves. Chakras are points where there is a particular accumulation of energy from the criss-crossing *nadis*—the energy pathways/vibrations—through which the prana, the cosmic energy, vitality, or life force flows. When the nadis are not flowing freely—when there are traffic jams on the energy pathways so to speak—energy can not then freely flow in and out of chakras.

In yoga, metabolism is closely connected with prana and is specifically linked to two "chakras," the purification chakra in the throat area, and the digestive/nourishment chakra in the navel area. According to Swami Rameshwarananda, there are several ways yoga can help someone with thyroid disease. But first, he has a word of caution:

> You can begin your practice of yoga as a way to improve your overall health, with a focus on your thyroid, but do not stop taking your thyroid medicine. Eventually, you may find that you need less medicine, or even, as some students have reported, be able to stop taking

your medicine entirely. But you should only change your medicine with your doctor's monitoring and supervision.

Swami Rameshwarananda recommends that people begin a program of basic yoga postures (exercises beneficial for everyone) that are designed to help harmonize the different bodies. These exercises are known as saraw hitta asanas and are best learned from an experienced yoga instructor. You can see them performed in a videotape demonstrated by Swami Rameshwarananda or learn similar exercises in a beginner's yoga class.

Penelope, a thirty-four-year-old with Hashimoto's thyroiditis, swears by her yoga exercises as the one thing that truly improves her health:

> I have been studying yoga for a little over a year and am much, much more flexible and stronger than before. I was diagnosed with fibromyalgia over two years ago, and since starting the yoga, I have no pain or fatigue at all. The yoga has also been wonderful for muscle aches, and it even helped my libido.

Next, Swami Rameshwarananda recommends the practice of pranayam (pran-a-YAM), the breathing exercises that help to cleanse and harmonize the nadi energy pathways and clear out obstructions—physical, mental, and emotional. Many yoga centers and alternative health workshops offer this training.

The most basic pranayam of all is deep abdominal breathing. To try it yourself, lay flat on your back, or stand. Put your hand on your abdomen and take a deep breath, filling your belly with air so your hand rises, then exhale. Start basic pranayam practice by simply doing this for ten or fifteen minutes each day, and you'll be surprised at how much more relaxed, yet energetic, you'll feel.

Third, there is a specific breathing exercise that is designed to help the thyroid and the throat chakra. Breathe in through your nose, focusing the inhalation toward the back of your throat. Your throat should feel slightly "closed" or "blocked" while you perform this breathing exercise. Mentally, you should try to feel as if you are taking in the air *through* the front of your throat. Do this

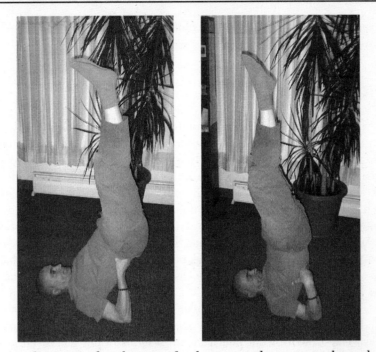

several times a day, but not for long periods, as it might make you dizzy.

Finally, there is a specific asana or pose that is thought to be of great benefit to the thyroid. The "half shoulder stand" (viparit karani mudra) and "shoulder stand" (sarvangasan) positions both invert and stimulate the thyroid. According to Swami Rameshwarananda, the shoulder stand is considered one of the most powerful positions in yoga, and in addition to helping the thyroid, it is thought to prolong life through its affect on the metabolism and pranic energy.

In a shoulder stand, you lie flat on your back, and keeping your legs together, you raise them up until they are at a right angle to your shoulders/neck, perpendicular to the floor, chin tucked into your chest, resting the weight of your body on your shoulders and elbows, arms supporting your hips. Work up to a daily session of a full two minutes by starting with two or three shorter sessions. Swami Rameshwarananda counsels that you should always stop and consult an experienced yoga instructor if doing a shoulder stand makes you feel dizzy, uncomfortable, or interferes with your breathing.

HOMEOPATHY

If you've seen a cold and flu remedy called Oscillococcinum on the drugstore shelf, you've seen contemporary homeopathic medicine in action. The current practice of homeopathy is based on the 200-year-old work of German doctor Samuel Hahnemann. His idea is that you can stimulate the immune system to fight illness by administering a homeopathic remedy—a microscopic, extremely diluted amount of an herb, mineral, or other substance—that would cause similar symptoms in a healthy person. The theory is "like cures like," similar to the concept behind giving a vaccine that contains some elements of the disease the vaccination is meant to prevent.

Homeopathy was very popular in the U.S. in the late 1800s, and nearly 15 percent of all physicians at that time used homeopathy. The growth of the pharmaceutical industry put almost all homeopaths out of business until recently, when the popularity of homeopathy has returned. Currently, there are an estimated 3,000 physicians and other healthcare personnel practicing homeopathy in the U.S., and many more practitioners in Europe, Canada, and throughout the world.

There are two different ways to pursue homeopathic treatment. The first is to visit a classical homeopath, who will conduct a lengthy interview about physical and psychological preferences and symptoms, and then recommend homeopathic remedies based on an analysis of the responses. The second is to use homeopathic formulas for particular ailments. Several brands are sold at health and vitamin stores.

Homeopathy is gaining in popularity, and some homeopaths say they are able to reverse or even heal hypothyroidism. I'll be honest. I've had great success using homeopathic remedies for allergies, cold, flu, and teething for myself and my family. On the basis of success with the individual remedies, I found a highly recommended classical homeopath to treat my hypothyroidism. Unfortunately, most of the thyroid remedies seemed to make me feel far worse for weeks on end, until I finally gave up.

I've talked to others who also have not had success with homeopathy for hypothyroidism. Prtha is another person who tried homeopathic medicine:

> While I was on the homeopathic medicine, the homeopathic doc had me cutting my Synthroid dose more and more, yet the homeopathic medicine was not sufficiently working and all my symptoms of hypothyroidism came back! Well, even now, on this inappropriate dose of Synthroid I am on, all symptoms are not gone, but they weren't as bad as on the homeopathic medicine!

I haven't heard from any people who have had success with homeopathy alone for their thyroid treatment. Rather, when they reported success, it was in conjunction with diet and nutritional support, making it impossible to isolate which treatment was responsible for the improvement. Perhaps homeopathy's success with thyroid is unique to each person or depends on the particular skill or the homeopath. I still feel that the jury is out on use of homeopathy for hypothyroidism.

However, according to medical studies, where homeopathy really shines, and where, as I mentioned, I had great success, as have others, is in dealing with conditions like hay fever, allergies, and migraines. Since many patients have worsening allergies due to hypothyroidism, homeopathic remedies may be of help in dealing with those specific symptoms.

If you are looking for a homeopath, be sure to find someone licensed to practice. There are a number of accreditations, including:.

• D.Ht. (Diplomate in Homeotherapeutics), which is given by the American Board of Homeotherapeutics to M.D.s and osteopaths who have practiced homeopathy for at least three years.

• C.C.H. (Certified in Classical Homeopathy), given by the Council for Homeopathic Certification.

- D.H.A.N.P. (Diplomate of the Homeopathic Academy of Naturopathic Physicians), given to naturopathic physicians who have completed at least 250 hours of homeopathic coursework and passed an exam.

AROMATHERAPY

Think about how the smell of vanilla, or your spouse's favorite cologne, or the scent of fresh pine can make you feel. That's basic aromatherapy—tapping into the ability of scent to affect emotions, and ultimately, health and body functions. Aromatherapy uses highly concentrated essential oils to evoke emotional and physical responses to heal the body. Essential oils can function as muscle relaxants, circulatory stimulants, hormone precursors, and can work to remove metabolic waste and enhance immunity. Researchers have recently found that aromatherapy can stimulate powerful relaxation responses, which in turn, increase immunity, so there is a scientific basis to aromatherapy. Aromatherapy oils are typically delivered via baths, diffusers (which heat the oil to evaporate it through a room), inhalation, massage, and topical use.

When it comes to aromatherapy for hypothyroidism, there are no specific studies relating aromatherapy to the thyroid itself. In terms of general health and energy, however, there are many things you can do with essential oils to improve your overall well-being. According to Mindy Green, aromatherapy and herbal expert at the Herb Research Foundation, two areas where aromatherapy can play a specific part are reducing stress and helping to support the adrenal system.

For stress and adrenal support, lavender, and the firs and pines, are good essential oils. Says Green:

> You can take three drops of lavender plus two drops of fir or pine to a teaspoon of vegetable oil, and add that to your nightly bath. Simply smelling lavender is a useful tonic for stress reduction and has been proven to increase alpha waves, the relaxing waves in the brain.

Green cautions that bath-and-body stores often carry synthetic or perfume-based oils. Be careful to use only plant-based oils, which are typically sold at health food stores and some specialty stores that specialize in good essential oils.

She also described how you could condition your brain to perceive a particular fragrance as a stress-reducer. According to Green:

> Fragrance is associated with emotion and hunger and appetite, so it's important that you pick a fragrance that you find pleasant but that doesn't have any associated memory. You need to then smell that aroma whenever you're feeling happy and relaxed. It might take you three weeks or so to actually "program and exercise" that part of your brain to recognize this aroma and associate it with relaxation. You'll find that when you go back to it when you're feeling stressed, it can then help trigger relaxation and reduce your stress.

Aromatherapy is also promising for weight loss. If you're interested in more about this, Green recommends looking into the work and books of Dr. Alan R. Hirsch of the Smell and Taste Treatment and Research Foundation in Chicago. Dr. Hirsch, a neurologist and psychiatrist, has published a book titled *Scentsational Weight Loss,* which describes how certain scents can satisfy the brain's hunger centers and stimulate weight loss. On a regular program of inhaling certain odors, Dr. Hirsch found that patients lost an average of 2.1 percent body mass per month or approximately five pounds per month.

✿　　✿　　✿

If you choose to pursue these or any other complementary or alternative therapies, be sure to keep your conventional doctors informed of what you're doing, or any herbs, supplements, or drugs you might be taking. By involving your conventional practitioners, you give them a partnership role in your wellness and can potentially avoid conflicts in treatments that might arise.

CHAPTER 8

Breaking New Ground: Answering the Question of T3

If everyone is thinking alike, then no one is thinking.
BENJAMIN FRANKLIN

Two health practitioners, 2,000 miles apart, enjoy consistent success treating thyroid patients who, after suffering years with various symptoms of hypothyroidism, become truly *well*. Both doctors swim against the current of popular medical opinion. They practice based on their own medical judgment and patients' needs, not according to standard doctrine. In their pioneering practices, they are finding the reasons behind routine underdiagnosis of hypothyroidism, and the solutions for many long-term unresolved symptoms.

This chapter looks at the work of Dr. Kenneth Blanchard, a conventionally trained internist/endocrinologist, and Dr. John Lowe, a pain management specialist who specializes in hypometabolic problems like fibromyalgia syndrome and hypothyroidism and who heads up the Fibromyalgia Research Foundation. Both doctors offer answers and solutions for patients who do not fit into the prevalent TSH level and levothyroxine-driven means of diagnosing and treating thyroid dysfunction. Both have found success using T3. And both have in part been proven right by the conventional T3 research reported in the *New England Journal of Medicine* in February of 1999.

Before we get into Dr. Blanchard and Dr. Lowe's treatments and ideas, and the findings of the *New England Journal* article, it's useful to take a look at the relationship between autoimmune hypothyroidism, fibromyalgia, and a third related problem, chronic fatigue syndrome (CFS).

OVERVIEW, SYMPTOMS, AND DIAGNOSIS

A fair percentage of people with autoimmune hypothyroidism end up also being diagnosed with fibromyalgia and/or CFS. And conversely, significant percentages of patients with fibromyalgia and CFS also have underlying thyroid imbalances. This raises a key question: what is the relationship among autoimmune hypothyroidism, fibromyalgia, and CFS, and are there common treatments to resolve these problems and the resulting symptoms?

Interestingly, many of the symptoms cross over to all three conditions. Exhaustion, fatigue, muscle cramps and pains, poor sleeping, depression, and lowered resistance to infections are common to the three conditions.

The primary complaint in fibromyalgia syndrome is the muscular and joint pain, a round-the-clock pain that rarely goes away. Fibromyalgia can be diagnosed by a detailed 18-point "tender point" examination.

For people with CFS, the main complaint is the unrelenting fatigue. Even the smallest physical exertion can put the sufferer in bed for days. There is no official clinical test to make a firm diagnosis of CFS. Instead, doctors typically rule out other underlying illnesses before making a CFS diagnosis.

With autoimmune hypothyroidism (Hashimoto's disease), symptoms are broader, including fatigue and exhaustion, depression, weight gain, hair loss, muscular and joint pain, excessive weight gain, dry hair and skin, hair loss, and menstrual irregularities.

Fibromyalgia strikes mostly women between the ages of 20 and 50. The majority of diagnosed cases of CFS occur in women, most 25 to 45 years old. And thyroid problems are known to affect women seven times more often than men, most frequently women in their adulthood.

CAUSES OF THE DISEASES

It's likely that there is some autoimmune component to fibromyalgia and CFS, as there is in autoimmune hypothyroidism. *The Journal of Clinical Investigation* found that approximately 52 percent of CFS patients develop autoantibodies indicative of autoimmune reactions. In a 1994 article reported in a German journal, a study of 375 patients with CFS showed an increased occurrence of auto-antibodies in the CFS patients, especially microsomal thyroid anti-bodies. According to the researchers, this suggests that "CFS is associated with or the beginning of manifest autoimmune disease."

There are many hypotheses as to the causes behind autoimmune diseases, but few answers. Researchers theorize that bacteria, viruses, toxins, and even some drugs may play a role in triggering an autoim-mune process in someone who already has a genetic, inherited predis-position to develop such a disorder. Some fibromyalgia researchers are looking at abnormally low levels of the hormone cortisol and its rela-tionship to fibromyalgia. Other fibromyaigia researchers are studying regulation of the adrenal gland (which makes cortisol) in fibromyalgia. Some medical researchers believe that a virus—such as Epstein-Barr, the mononucleosis virus—is at the core of these diseases. And while no single virus or cause has been firmly associated with CFS, fi-bromyalgia, or autoimmune thyroid disease, one medical journal reported that 78 percent of the CFS patients studied in one re-search effort also tested positive for the Epstein-Barr virus.

Anecdotally, many thyroid patients report having had serious bouts of mononucleosis, or recurrent Epstein-Barr virus, prior to being diagnosed with their thyroid problem. Other researchers point to an accident (such as an auto accident) or other trauma that activates the immune system. The immune system, which ordinarily returns to normal after successfully fighting an infection, then re-mains in a hyperactive state.

The fact that many autoimmune diseases affect women in far greater numbers than men also brings up the question of a hor-monal component, another issue that is being studied. Practitioners like Dr. Elizabeth Vliet, for example, believe that the high inci-dence of hypothyroidism and fibromylagia in women points to the need to study the ovarian hormonal aspects of these conditions.

ARE FIBROMYALGIA, CFS, AND AUTOIMMUNE HYPOTHYROIDISM THE SAME ILLNESS?

Some doctors and health practitioners theorize that CFS, fibromy-algia, and autoimmune hypothyroidism are really all variations of the same or similar autoimmune dysfunction, and the primary difference is the chief symptom for each sufferer. Interestingly, this is the theory held by both Drs. Blanchard and Lowe, who both have a successful record treating patients with hypothyroidism and/or fibromyalgia. Both believe that the use of T3 is absolutely essential to the success of their therapies.

While Drs. Lowe and Blanchard have different philosophies and treatment protocols, their success depends on using T3 in varying forms. They both argue that TSH "normal ranges" are not, in fact, a reliable measurement of what is normal for some people, either due to too wide a range or due to the TSH test's inability to detect underlying hypothyroidism. Underlying hypothyroidism can occur when there is peripheral or cellular resistance to thyroid hormone, or insufficient or impaired T4 to T3 conversion.

Pituitary "general" resistance to thyroid hormone (known by its acronym RTH) is a rare disease. So when people suggest to their doctors, "Maybe I am resistant to thyroid hormone," doctors usually are quick to dismiss it. However, problems of peripheral or cellular resistance to thyroid hormone and inability to convert T4 to T3 properly may well explain the success of Drs. Lowe and Blanchard's therapies. This is why I believe it is important for those of you with unrelieved symptoms and "normal TSH values" to thoroughly investigate what these two doctors have to say and consider whether or not to pursue these types of treatment approaches for your own hypothyroidism.

Kenneth Blanchard, M.D.—"The Answer is in the Proper Balance of T3 to T4"

Kenneth Blanchard, M.D., has an internal medicine and endocrinology practice in Newton Lower Falls, Massachusetts. He came to my attention because I kept receiving emails from thyroid patients, nominating him to be included in my Web site's "Thyroid Top Docs" listing. So many people wrote saying that even after years of suffering with hypothyroidism, they'd had success being treated by Dr. Blanchard, I decided to talk to him myself.

Dr. Blanchard is one physician who is out to tackle "The Many Myths of Hypothyroidism," which is, not coincidentally, the title of his forthcoming book. It turns out that, in years of dealing with hypothyroid patients, Dr. Blanchard has discovered a number of myths that he believes leave many people unable to live well with hypothyroidism because they are simply not being treated properly.

Dr. Blanchard feels that one particularly prevalent myth is the idea that "normal" blood tests can rule out hypothyroidism in individuals with a very strong history, family history, and physical findings suggestive of the disorder. This is a myth, according to Dr. Blanchard, because the normal ranges of the tests are so wide and people at the end of the ranges are often excluded from valid diagnoses:

> What doctors are always told is that the TSH test gives us a yes-or-no answer. In fact, I think that's fundamentally wrong. The pituitary TSH is controlled, not just by how much T4 and T3 is in circulation, but T4 is getting converted to T3 at the pituitary level. Excess T3 generated at the pituitary level can falsely suppress TSH.

Dr. Blanchard is suggesting that while TSH levels may be low, the body itself is responding and reacting as if TSH is much higher, thus creating a situation of hypothyroidism.

He also believes that it is a myth that all patients are adequately treated for hypothyroidism on levothyroxine alone. He has found this is not the case for many of his patients, who have suffered years of poor health from hypothyroidism, despite treatment.

Dr. Blanchard has developed a very specific method of determining the proper ratio of synthetic T4 and T3 needed to achieve what he calls a "proper physiologic dose of thyroid hormone," a dose that resolves many of the ongoing symptoms and problems. He uses a specially compounded form of T3, which he adds to standard levothyroxine therapy, resulting in significant improvements in many patients he sees.

> The fundamental reason for using T3 is that we know that the normal secretion of the thyroid gland includes primarily T4 and a smaller amount of T3. When we give small amounts of T3 along with T4, we're simply reproducing the normal physiology better.

Dr. Blanchard is very specific that it must be a very small dosage of T3, which he calculates and calibrates very specifically, in order to avoid having too much or too little T3 in the system. He has not had successful results using the drug Thyrolar, because, as he sees it, the percentage of T3 in Thyrolar is simply too high.

Dr. Blanchard is also not a proponent of natural thyroid. Some practitioners prefer natural products like Armour because they are reported to have other components besides T3 and T4, elements like "T1 and T2." Proponents claim this is why natural thyroid works better for some people than levothyroxine, or even levothyroxine plus T3:

> I've explored the issue of Armour in great detail. Armour is approximately 80 percent T4 and 20 percent T3 and 20 percent is too much T3. But to see if the other elements of Armour, like T1 and T2, made a difference, I've even gone to the point of having my compounding pharmacist actually add pure T4 thyroid extract to Armour to get better T4/T3 ratios. I tried it personally, some patients tried it as well, and there wasn't anything particularly better about it.

For Dr. Blanchard, the most fundamental determinant of how tissues function thyroid-wise is the proper balance between T4 and T3 at the tissue level. He believes the majority is best served by treatment with proportions of T4 and T3 that reproduce the normal physiology. This means a regimen where the T3 dose amounts to roughly 2 percent to 5 percent of the T4 dose.

Dr. Blanchard believes that in order to live well with hypothyroidism, patients must have their underlying thyroid problem properly treated:

> When we get the people I treat on a pretty good dosage, including the T3 time-release capsule, most of them can't believe how much better they are. Many of them have almost sadness once the burden of hypothyroidism is released off of them, and they realize how many years of their lives they existed carrying this anchor around with them.

Dr. Blanchard believes that fibromyalgia results from underlying hypothyroidism, and that ultimately, the underlying thyroid problem must be addressed to resolve these symptoms. In the case of fibromyalgia symptoms in particular, Dr. Blanchard feels that T4 alone is particularly ineffective, and the use of small doses of T3 becomes absolutely essential to effective treatment.

Detailed explanations of Dr. Blanchard's theories and ideas are set out fully in his forthcoming book, *The Many Myths of Hypothyroidism*. For more information about the book, you can contact Dr. Blanchard's office, 2000 Washington Street, Suite 565, Newton Lower Falls, MA 02462, 617-527-1810.

John Lowe, DC—TSH Suppression and T3 are the Solutions

Dr. Lowe, an innovative researcher who heads the Fibromyalgia Research Foundation, comes to the issue of hypothyroidism and its treatment questioning what he describes as the four conventional endocrinology mandates:

> (1) The only cause of thyroid hormone deficiency symptoms is hypo-thyroidism; (2) only patients with hypothyroidism "according to lab results" should be permitted to use thyroid hormone; (3) the hypothy-roid patient should be allowed to use only T4; and (4) the patient's dosage should not suppress the TSH level.

Dr. Lowe has challenged these preconceptions as part of his long-standing effort to learn more about treatment-resistant fibromyalgia. The result is a treatment protocol based on his findings that the unresolved symptoms associated with treated hypothyroidism and fi-bromyalgia are often evidence of untreated or undertreated hypothy-roidism, or partial cellular resistance to thyroid hormone.

A unique aspect of Dr. Lowe's theories is his recognition that a patient with cellular resistance may have perfectly normal circulating thyroid hormone levels yet have the symptoms and signs of hypothy-roidism. I believe this is an important aspect of Dr. Lowe's treatments that may point to the reason for his success. He has found, however, from his discussions with other fibromyalgia/CFS researchers that most are unaware of such potential mechanisms. He says:

> To them, if a patient has a normal TSH level, and especially if the patient's symptoms don't improve with replacement dosages of T4,

her condition cannot possibly be related in any way to thyroid hormone. Recent scientific research, however, has shown this belief to be false.

If you have autoimmune hypothyroidism, it's fairly common to develop some classic fibromyalgia symptoms, such as muscle/joint pain, aches, and sleep disturbances. According to Dr. Lowe, the conventional physician is likely to consider any new or worsened symptoms as evidence that there's yet another condition—such as fibromyalgia—*in addition* to the autoimmune thyroid problem. To Dr. Lowe, however, that means that the newly developing symptoms may be evidence of undertreated hypothyroidism:

> As thyroid hormone deficiency worsens, the number of tissues involved and the severity of the resulting symptoms increase. The patient typically experiences the worsening deficiency as an increased number of symptoms of greater severity. In most cases, such patients simply need a more appropriate dosage or form of thyroid hormone to recover from all their symptoms.

Dr. Lowe believes that rigid adherence to the so-called "normal range" does not show whether a patient has enough circulating T3 to maintain normal metabolism in cells. His research shows that safe, but suppressive, doses are often more effective at eliminating associated health problems that are of greatest concern. T4 to T3 conversion can be impaired, so the fact that a patient has a normal TSH level does not mean that her tissue metabolism is normal.

According to Dr. Lowe, one study showed that replacement dosages of thyroid hormone—dosages that keep the TSH within the normal range—mildly lowered patients' high cholesterol levels, but TSH-suppressive dosages further lowered the levels significantly.

Many published reports and our studies show that the TSH level does not correlate with various tests of tissue metabolism. Dr. Lowe feels this is important because making tissue metabolism normal should be the goal of all treatment with hypothyroid patients. When the hypothyroid patient is restricted to a dosage of T4 that keeps the TSH within the normal range, testing will produce evidence of abnormal metabolism in multiple tissues.

Dr. Lowe has found that TSH-suppressive dosages of thyroid hormone can also reduce a patients' risk for disease. Dr. Lowe finds that lower dosages of thyroid hormone have been found to be associated with progression of coronary atherosclerosis and higher dosages (including TSH-suppressive dosages) associated with a halting of the progression. In his studies, Dr. Lowe has extensively tested patients and determined that there is nothing harmful to patients in having their TSH suppressed by these dosages of thyroid hormone. Dr. Lowe sees the far greater danger being the clear adverse consequences of undertreated resistance, resulting in conditions such as fibromyalgia, CFS, and liver and cardiovascular diseases.

Dr. Lowe believes the hypothyroid patient has two options: She can submit to using a replacement dosage of thyroid hormone and remain symptomatic, thus risking premature death from cardiovascular disease. Or she can find a physician who will completely ignore her TSH level and find a dosage that produces normal tissue metabolism.

Some researchers dismiss thyroid hormone replacement as a possible treatment for fibromyalgia symptoms or CFS. According to Dr. Lowe, however, "replacement" as defined by these researchers typically doesn't work because replacement means the use of only T4 to keep the TSH within normal range, and that is simply not enough to free most hypothyroid patients from their symptoms. The assumption that replacement dosages of T4 are the only acceptable treatment prevents other researchers from seeing the mechanism of most patients' fibromyalgia/CFS—inadequate thyroid hormone regulation of tissues.

Dr. Lowe believes that the combination of T4 and T3 generally works better than T4 alone with hypothyroid patients, and in some cases T3 alone works best. Dr. Lowe found that when hypothyroid patients were treated with T4 first, gradually increasing the dosage, if it didn't provide much benefit or any at all, patients were switched to T3. Many patients do not benefit from the use of T4, regardless of how high the dosage.

> T4 alone is a poor option for many hypothyroid fibromyalgia patients, and it is useless for fibromyalgia patients with cellular resistance to thyroid hormone. Most of these patients, who make up about 44 percent

of the fibromyalgia patient population according to our studies, benefit only from very large dosages of T3. Only a minority of hypothyroid fibromyalgia patients satisfactorily improved with the use of T4 alone. In contrast, T3 alone almost always enables patients to improve or recover.

According to Dr. Lowe, T3 works because many patients have both hypothyroidism and cellular resistance to thyroid hormone, and these patients do not benefit from T4 or natural thyroid, even with the relatively large amount of T3 in desiccated thyroid. Dr. Lowe finds that virtually all resistance patients benefit only from large dosages of synthetic T3, far more than desiccated thyroid provides.

We have shown conclusively that these patients have cellular resistance to thyroid hormone, and we have shown that they become normal (without any evidence of overstimulation) only with as much as twice or more T3 than the typical hypothyroid patient without tissue resistance requires to get well. Our findings confirm those of other researchers in the 1950s and early 1960s. These researchers reported that many patients improved or recovered from their hypothyroid-like symptoms and low metabolic rates with T3 after failing to benefit from even large dosages of T4 or desiccated thyroid.

Many researchers express concerns that the use of T3 alone is somehow not safe. However, according to Dr. Lowe, patients have recovered with T3 and have remained recovered for fifteen years or so without any adverse effects whatsoever:

And when I say no adverse effects, I base that on objective testing that shows no such effects. The only drawback I've found to using T3 is a social one: it is harder for patients to get their doctors to prescribe T3 in the dosages they need.

Dr. Lowe's opinions contradict the conventional thought now prevalent amongst mainstream medical practitioners that the TSH test and synthetic T4 treatments are the sole answer to diagnosing and managing hypothyroidism. Dr. Lowe believes that the pressure to conform to the consensus view has created a culture where physicians who use an accepted method of diagnosis or treatment are praised, even if the method did little or nothing for patients. He also believes that physicians are condemned or even blackballed if they use an "unaccepted" form of diagnosis or treatment, even if that method helps patients.

Dr. Lowe also finds that medicine has become characterized by what he calls "extremist medical technocracy," an excessive reliance on the results of technological measures, such as blood tests. At the same time, we're seeing the disappearance of clinical medicine, the type of medicine that relies on the clinician's opinion of the patient's history, symptoms, and signs—in combination with test results.

Dr. Lowe is also concerned by two additional factors that have contributed to this environment: defensive medical practice, and the big business of medicine. According to Dr. Lowe, physicians can best legally protect themselves when they can defend their diagnostic and treatment decisions with the results of objective tests, test results that are approved by the conventional medical establishment. TSH tests are a source of income for thyroid researchers who developed the tests, companies that produce and market the tests, medical laboratories that provide them, and physicians who order them. This economic motivation is a powerful force in maintaining various practices in medicine.

Dr. Lowe makes some excellent points, and his understanding of both medicine and the politics of medicine make his assessments and recommendations particularly relevant. In this book, I can't possibly provide the in-depth analysis of the various issues—including diagnosis, treatment, and detailed studies showing results and outcomes—that support Dr. Lowe's ideas. This is something covered in Dr. Lowe's own book, *The Metabolic Treatment of Fibromyalgia*, which I highly recommend.

THE T3 RESEARCH AND CONTROVERSY

In February of 1999, the *New England Journal of Medicine* published a research report that has the potential to revolutionize the face of thyroid hormone treatment and the quality of life of many people with hypothyroidism. The article, "Effects of Thyroxine as Compared with Thyroxine plus Triiodothyronine in Patients with

Hypothyroidism," reported that adding T3 (triiodothyronine) to the standard T4 therapy improved the quality of life for most hypothyroid patients. Essentially, researchers took a group of 33 people who were hypothyroid, either due to autoimmune thyroid disease or removal of their thyroids due to thyroid cancer. All the patients were studied for two five-week periods. During one five-week period, the patient received his or her regular dose of levothyroxine (T4) alone. During the other five-week period, the patient received T4 *plus* triiodothyronine (T3.) In the T4 plus T3 phase, 50 µg of the patient's typical levothyroxine dose was replaced by 12.5 µg of triiodothyronine (T3). A variety of blood, cognitive, mood, and physical tests were conducted at various stages of research.

From the standpoint of physiological effects, the differences between pulse, blood pressure, reflexes, and a variety of other functions for T4 alone, versus T4 plus T3, were very small. Blood pressure and cholesterol, in fact, dropped slightly on the T4 plus T3. Results were dramatic, however, were in mental functioning. All the patients performed better on a variety of standard neuropsychological tasks when taking the T4 plus T3. Patients' psychological state also showed improvement on T4 plus T3. At the end of the study, patients were asked whether they preferred the first or second treatments. Twenty patients said they preferred the T4 plus T3 treatment, eleven had no preference either way, and only two preferred T4 only. The twenty patients who preferred T4 plus T3 reported that they had more energy, improved concentration, and just felt better overall.

The researchers also recommended the ideal thyroid hormone replacement program for someone without a thyroid gland or whose thyroid gland is nearly nonfunctioning: "10 µg of triiodothyronine daily in sustained-release form . . . along with enough thyroxine to ensure euthyroidism."

This study has major implications for people who don't feel well on their current thyroid hormone replacement.

- If you are on standard levothyroxine-only therapy, it's possible that, like the majority of study subjects, you too could feel better with the addition of T3 in the recommended dosage ratio.
- If you are on Armour Thyroid, Westhroid, Naturethroid, or Thyrolar, the current percentages of T3 in those drugs *may* be

somewhat too high for you, compared to the recommended ratios described in this study. Optimal results may be obtained by modifying the treatment regimen to conform more specifically to the recommended ratio the researchers described.

This is groundbreaking research, finally confirming in the research environment what many patients, myself included, and some doctors have been claiming for a number of years: Levothyroxine-only thyroid hormone replacement does not leave a substantial percentage of hypothyroid patients feeling well, and these patients feel and function better when T3 is added to their thyroid hormone replacement. Interestingly, this research also offers an explanation for why patients have felt well all along on alternative thyroid drugs like the natural Armour Thyroid, Westhroid and Naturethroid, which contain T4 and T3 naturally, and the synthetic T4/T3 drug Thyrolar.

If you are on thyroid hormone replacement and don't feel well, I recommend that you notify your doctor about this research study and get a copy of this article for yourself as well. You can visit this book's Web site for a link to online ordering of the article from the *New England Journal of Medicine*, or go to its Web site at *http://www.nejm.org* or call 1-800-THE-NEJM and order a copy to be faxed or mailed for $10. Ask for "Effects of Thyroxine as Compared with Thyroxine plus Triiodothyronine in Patients with Hypothyroidism," Volume 340, Issue 6. You can also get a copy at many libraries.

Will the Medical Community Adopt the Findings?

Though patients might assume that such exciting news about improved treatment would be applauded by the medical community, the real story is quite different. Anything that challenges the status quo meets serious resistance from the slow-to-change medical establishment. Additionally, pharmaceutical companies are bound to poke holes in any research that could potentially challenge the market for the levothyroxine products they sell.

The editorial that accompanied the *New England Journal of Medicine* article reveals a closing of the ranks, giving a clear picture of what the party line is according to the old guard endocrinology community. In it, thyroidologist Dr. Anthony D. Toft, of the Royal

Infirmary, Edinburgh, Scotland expressed the opinion that physicians should not add the T3 hormone to the treatment until study findings are confirmed by additional research. One reason for Toft's assertion is, as he claims: "most, if not all, of the currently available combined preparations of thyroid hormones contain an excess of triiodothyronine as compared with thyroxine."

To say that this is a reason not to use T3 in treatment is highly illogical. It is true that Thyrolar and the natural T4/T3 products have a higher percentage of T3 than the researchers used in their study. But Cytomel, a T3-only drug, is readily available, and compounding pharmacies almost anywhere can easily prepare time-released T3. The vast majority of people with hypothyroidism are already on conventional levothyroxine treatment. It would be a simple matter of adding compounded time-released T3, which is what the researchers recommended, or Cytomel in proper proportions.

Toft also argues that the majority of patients taking thyroxine "have no complaints about their medication." Here, I would ask what research Toft is quoting. I don't believe there is any. Toft's opinion actually directly contradicts the findings of informal research conducted by the Thyroid Foundation of America that showed that the majority of post-Graves' disease hypothyroid patients still suffered a variety of symptoms when on levothyroxine.

It's baffling why, in the face of notable improvement in function, and little evidence of any detrimental physical effects, doctors like Toft would rather wait for more research, instead of treat patients more effectively. But then Dr. Toft himself has been quite an active proponent of the "normal range constitutes treatment" and "low-normal TSH is dangerous" philosophies of hypothyroid management that have left so many countless millions of patients undiagnosed, undertreated, or maltreated.

Toft's analyses, opinions, interpretations, and editorials have, according to Dr. John Lowe, played an instrumental role in the sad plight of hypothyroid patients today:

> If we were to hold a Nuremberg trial to decide who to hold guilty for subjecting untold millions of hypothyroid patients to a low quality of life, suicidal depression, progressive cardiovascular disease, and premature death—all from too little thyroid hormone tissue regula-

tion—I would vote to include Toft as a defendant. He is one of the thyroidologists who back in the 1980s began using the term "TSH-suppressive T4 dosages" as synonymous with "thyrotoxicosis" in the research literature. To consider TSH-suppressive dosages as synonymous with tissue thyrotoxicosis was clearly a false inference; it is one that has had disastrous consequences for the population of hypothyroid patients.

At a 1999 meeting on endocrinology at the University of California, San Francisco (UCSF), several doctors were already arguing against T3 therapy. Francis Greenspan, M.D., chief of the UCSF Thyroid Clinic, said that "patients respond beautifully to T4." Dr. Peter Yeo, a professor of medicine at UCSF, said that the use of T3 is unproven, and would not be advocated.

According to Dr. Lowe, the beliefs of doctors like these have become the prevailing doctrine.

Today, conventional physicians shiver in their shoes when they see a suppressed TSH level, even though the patient's TSH-suppressive dosage—and only that dosage—has gotten him or her well. So, at the physician's command, down goes the dosage and so, too, the health of the patient.

Meanwhile, if doctors like Toft, Greenspan, Yeo and their colleagues have their way, patients may wait forever for the big enough, long-enough, peer-reviewed-enough study that proves what the research has already shown, and patients already know.

Thyroid patients have wasted enough valuable time not feeling well, living lives at half-speed, waiting to feel better, while doctors tell us that more research is needed. They could literally research our lives away. We already have the research findings that can help many people. And we have the anecdotal knowledge of thousands upon thousands of thyroid patients and their doctors who are able to live well with the use of T3 drugs. Thyroid patients have waited long enough. Responsible doctors owe it to their patients to carefully consider whether or not T3 therapy will benefit their patients.

In Our Voices

"On Being Thoughtless" —Marge's Story

About three years ago, I realized that I was becoming an incredibly thoughtless person. I don't mean overlooking the niceties of saying "please" or "thank you," or neglecting to send birthday cards. I mean not having any conscious thoughts, ideas, or opinions. Whether chatting with friends, family, or colleagues, I simply didn't know what to say or how to say it. I felt very puzzled most of the time and was becoming uncharacteristically quiet.

By day, I work with children who have communication disorders. I teach them how to understand what they hear around them, how to synthesize their own thoughts and ideas, and how to express themselves using clear and fluent speech. Before I became thoughtless, in my free time I wrote restaurant and movie reviews for a community monthly, finished most of the *New York Times* Sunday crossword puzzle regularly, and played a killer game of Scrabble. I read three or four books a week and the *Washington Post* daily. My world was words.

Initially, I assumed it was stress. So, annoyed with the inconvenience of it all, I promised myself that I would slow down and smell the roses. Waiting for my self-sacrifice to pay off, I attempted to subdue my internal confusion by relying on external cues to keep me in conversational loops. I waited until someone asked me a direct question or until I noted polite facial expressions being flashed in my direction. Then I knew it was my turn to participate.

Sometimes, I began a response and verbal-mazed my way around, hoping to bump into what I really wanted to say. I usually figured out that I was making no sense at all by the (politely) pained expressions on listeners' faces.

I also started forgetting unusual things. I knew exactly where my keys and glasses were at all times. I hadn't lost my car in a parking lot in years. But one day, I argued with a colleague about an important parent conference we cancelled because some of the required paperwork was missing. She claimed that I had volunteered to do it and I insisted that I hadn't even attended the planning session. "How could I possibly be responsible for this miserable failure of a meeting?" I asserted loudly. Then, she showed me the sign-in roster for that planning session. My signature was on it.

A week later a principal-trainee called me into her office and expressed concern about my abilities to handle the responsibilities and pressures of my demanding job. She suggested that I might want to contact the Employee's Assistance Program. She cooed warmly, "Going for help is nothing to be ashamed of." I let her know, in a very direct, cold voice that after twenty years, I was able to do the job just fine. I delivered a knee-jerk thanks-for-your-concern and stormed out of her office, firmly slamming the door behind me.

I was truly alarmed about what was happening to me. I could no longer read a book or see a movie and recall the plot. I couldn't stay focused long enough for even a mediocre game of Scrabble and did only bits and pieces of the Sunday crossword puzzle. I had outbursts of tears when I didn't feel sad, muscular aches and pains when I hadn't been exercising, a skin rash that seemed to mysteriously come and go, and a constant case of shivers and chills no matter what the weather and no matter how many layers of clothing I wore. I rarely felt hungry and lost close to thirty pounds. When I looked in the mirror, I was frightened by the sallow face that surrounded my dark-rimmed vacant stare. But, the change that was the most disturbing to me was the slow, seemingly relentless thoughtlessness.

More than thirty years ago, my mother had become fairly thoughtless, and, by my senior year of high school, only vaguely resembled the vibrant woman who had been a high school varsity basketball player, the first woman graduate from Julliard with a major in double bass and one of the more attractive members of the trendy all-girl dance band she toured with in the late '30s. After she met and married my father, a fellow musician, she stopped touring and worked for agencies that supported their liberal politics and anti-McCarthyism beliefs. My grandmother had saved a news photo of her in the crowd of protesters at Union Square.

But the mother who is etched into my anxious heart is the woman who read the same page in the same book for several weeks before I couldn't stand it anymore and I made her turn the page. She started printing when she wrote to my older sister in college; she couldn't remember all the cursive forms. She generously offered to type my term papers for school, happily transforming them into gibberish. I secretly hand-wrote them back into English before passing them in. Somewhere between my sophomore and junior year, the constant drone of TV game shows replaced Bach, Beethoven, and Brahms on the stereo. My mother was not yet fifty.

Shortly after I turned fifty, at the beginning of October, I caught a cold and was still coughing with much discomfort and pain at the end of November. Two ten-day courses of antibiotics brought no relief and two sets of healthy lab results compelled my internist to imply that it might be psychosomatic. I angrily told her that I was going to find another doctor who was better trained in diagnostics than she seemed to be and exited in a huff.

But I didn't do that. Instead, I decided that I had the flu and that it just had to run its course, with the help of acupuncture, herbs and vitamins, quarts of juice, and gallons of hot tea. At home, my family was increasingly distraught about my failing health and I promised my partner that I would discuss it during what was usually a pro forma annual checkup with the gynecologist.

At that appointment in mid-January, the doctor, who had known me for ten years, immediately expressed concern about my unhealthy appearance. I mentioned the symptoms that I could remember and she murmured something about menopause and depression. I declined the prescriptions for Premarin and Prozac and snapped at her that the only thing I was depressed about was feeling so physically awful. They drew blood and sent me off for my mammogram. Later that week, her secretary called to say all the results were normal.

By the middle of February, I had used up all my sick leave by either coming in late or going home early. By now, I was also worried about driving. Two changes of bifocals had not corrected my blurry vision and my reflexes were dangerously slow in response to red lights. I decided to see a neurologist.

I sobbed throughout the entire interview, confessing that I had resisted coming to see him for months because my mother had died of Alzheimer's and now I had it, too. I told him about my musical childhood and that I could no longer clap my hands in time to music or sing on key. He patted my hand kindly and said something about what happens when women turn fifty. He also suggested that I see a mental health professional. I didn't answer because I was too busy hating myself for crying. The technician drew blood and the doctor did the exam. Later that week, his office called to say all the results were normal, but the doctor still wanted to schedule a follow-up.

Eight weeks later, in April, I watched him thumb through my chart looking for the lab results. My mind wandered as I struggled to pay attention. "That's odd," he said, finding them. "One of these thyroid levels is a little high. But I don't think it means anything. The other two are fine." This was the first lab report that had even hinted at an abnormal finding and I was suddenly alert with hope. "Can I have a copy of that?" He shrugged, "Sure," pronounced me healthy and sent me home with my copy of the report.

Following a two-hour nap, I sat down at the computer. Many clicks later and with my partner's guidance, I had surfed my way to a site for doctors. We waded through a professional article about the diagnosis and treatment of hypothyroidism. I skimmed most of the material because I couldn't read or understand most of the words. We highlighted the long list of symptoms that applied to me but only one sentence in the section on treatment: "the next step is a therapeutic trial of thyroid hormone." I scanned the list of eleven authors and miraculously recognized the last name. Some-one I knew years ago had seen this doctor and thought she was wonderful. My partner found her number and made an appoint-ment for me. Then I took another nap. Two weeks later, I handed the endocrinologist my highlighted copy of her article and my coveted lab report. I watched her quickly scan the neon-colored sentences. She ushered me into the examining room, listened to my heart and took my pulse, hammered at my knees and elbows, and waited a long time for them to jerk. She shook her head in disbelief, smiled and extended her hand. "Congratulations! I wholeheartedly agree with your diagnosis!"

For almost two years now, my hormone-deprived tissues have gratefully absorbed my daily dose of Synthroid. That nasty flu is finally gone, and my skin is its regular color sans rash. My body has been restored to its healthier Rubenesque shape. I am no longer abnormally cold and happily complained about the heat all summer long. My memory is slowly but steadily improving; I no longer need to carry a memo pad just to get through an ordinary day. I have attempted crossword puzzles again and recently played a fair game of Scrabble. My nightstand has six books awaiting my attention.

I still have episodes of breathing difficulties, blurry vision, and morning fatigue. I can usually manage to keep the bouts of unexplained moodiness to myself without offending anyone or embarrassing myself. Also, I am still plagued with muscular pain. But I'm optimistic that these too, shall pass.

I've been thinking a lot about my mother lately, and my family's notion that she had Alzheimer's disease. By the time she died in 1984 at the age of sixty-six, she looked and acted older than her healthy eight-six-year-old mother. As my own thoughts and words have returned, I've wondered about why, with all the information that is available about Alzheimer's these days, I've never heard anything mentioned about the physical changes my mother experienced. Her beautiful nails, always perfectly manicured, started to split and crack. Her hands and feet were icy cold to the touch. Her skin became very dry and her hair thinned out to the point of baldness. She complained that her vision was blurry, even with new bifocals. She slept late into the morning and took two or three naps a day. As she deteriorated, she and my grandmother, who had always had a warm and loving relationship, bickered constantly and screamed at each other frequently. She ate very little, and became dangerously thin, drawn, and brittle. She looked like a dried out twig, ready to snap.

I don't know if she went to a doctor or if family members intervened and tried to help; in our family, children were not included in adult discussions and decisions. After she died, I decided that she had gone for help because to think otherwise was more than I could bear. So I have fantasized about what she must have tried to explain to the doctor. Perhaps the doctor said that all women about her age start to notice differences as they approach "the Change," and that he could prescribe Premarin. If that had happened, I imagine that she might have told him that she had worked for Planned Parenthood for fifteen years as a young woman, knew all about menopause, and this was not it. Maybe the doctor asked her if she went out much socially since her husband's death. After all, he might have said, you're still a young, attractive woman. She might have tried to explain to him that she was scared about what was happening to her. He might have said, "There, there don't worry, Pearl. You're just under too much stress without Bob here to help you raise the girls. Why don't you take a little vacation?"

The family photos of my mom document her transformation from a Joan Crawford look-alike to a wizened old crazy-lady at 66. My endocrinologist has offered to look at them with me, but I'm afraid to bring them to her, afraid to get confirmation that my mother's life might have been spared, save for the daily routine of taking one little pill.

I still miss my mother. I cannot yet rid myself of the notion that she might have been treated thoughtlessly.

Marge Tolchin

PART III

SPECIAL CONCERNS OF HYPOTHYROIDISM

CHAPTER 9

Losing Weight Despite Hypothyroidism

I've been on a diet for two weeks and all I've lost is two weeks.
TOTIE FIELDS

I hear from hundreds of people each week who are desperately unhappy. Brides who want to fit into wedding dresses, new mothers who can't shed the baby weight, women who aren't willing to give up feeling fit and attractive, men who don't understand why their usual workout routine or daily runs aren't keeping the weight off anymore. People like me who have a closet filled with different sized clothing, reflecting different stages of a thyroid problem. We all are looking to answer one question: "How do I get rid of the weight???"

It's the number one complaint of people with hypothyroidism. For many of us, hypothyroidism is synonymous with the weight battle, and it's impossible even to separate the two problems in our minds. A hypothyroidism diagnosis is only the beginning of what becomes a lifelong battle with weight, all the while being told by doctors that weight gain or difficulty losing has *nothing* to do with thyroid disease.

I totally disagree!

Losing weight is not easy for many people with thyroid disease. It's a slow process, a far more difficult task than it is for people without metabolic problems. It is also a problem that has caused me, and *millions* of others, far more heartache than nearly any other aspect of hypothyroidism.

The good news is, there are answers, and there are solutions, so let's take a look at the issue of how hypothyroidism can play a role in weight problems, and what can be done to maintain a healthy weight with hypothyroidism.

WEIGHT PROBLEMS:
A SYMPTOM OF HYPOTHYROIDISM?

Occasionally, people who are hypothyroid will lose excessive weight, but that is uncommon. Typically, inappropriate weight gain—or the inability to lose weight despite rigorous diet and exercise—signals the onset of hypothyroidism. Does a weight problem mean you are hypothyroid? Chances are it doesn't. Only a percentage of weight problems are due to hypothyroidism.

Weight gain is often the first symptom to tip you off that there is a thyroid problem, but it often must be followed by other symptoms before doctors take it seriously. Claudia experienced this:

> I was 115 pounds, and then I started noticing that I was gaining weight and trying to lose I kept gaining. Tried everything from Nutri-System to joining exercise class. I still had energy, but I was becoming depressed. Finally, I thought I was losing my mind. They put me on Prozac. It still didn't help. I started being so tired. I continued gaining weight and was up to 140 pounds. So tired I couldn't put one foot in front of the other. People noticed I was so swollen in my face. Started with a terrible constipation I have never before had. I went to the doctor and asked him to run a test for thyroid. He did and it was very high.

Even if you ask specifically for a thyroid test, there are three reasons you might have some difficulty getting a doctor to test your thyroid, based on "weight gain" as your primary symptom. First, you're touching on some sensitive ground for doctors. In the past, some doctors prescribed thyroid hormone as a "diet" aid, even in the absence of any other evidence of a thyroid problem. Much like doctors don't typically prescribe amphetamines ("speed") for dieting anymore, they don't use thyroid hormone for weight loss anymore, and it's considered an outdated and potentially dangerous treatment.

Second, eating too much and not getting enough exercise is statistically far more likely to be the cause of a weight problem than a malfunctioning thyroid. Doctors fear that we are always looking for a scapegoat for unwanted weight gain. They're afraid that it's too easy for us to blame being overweight on a thyroid or "glandular" problem instead of addressing the real cause: eating too much and not exercising enough. This makes some doctors overly cautious about testing for, much less diagnosing, hypothyroidism.

When forty-five year-old Celia with undiagnosed hypothyroidism complained of weight gain, her doctor told her she needed to diet and exercise more:

> I was already walking forty minutes a day, five days a week, and not eating excessively, yet gaining weight all the time. Even though I always ate less than anyone else at table, I gained weight. I figured it was just "old age"—that after you reach forty this was inevitable. I thought maybe I needed to exercise even more. . . .

Third, even if you protest that you are rigorously dieting and exercising, doctors may be rightfully skeptical. People often underestimate their total food, calorie, or fat intake, or overstate the amount and intensity of their workouts. It's not irrational for a doctor to assume that the typical person's idea of a diet is probably not sufficiently low-calorie or lowfat, and an exercise program not sufficiently strenuous, to lose weight.

To help counteract any resistance your doctor may have about testing your thyroid, be sure to bring your Hypothyroid Checklist with you so you can make sure your doctor is aware of your hypothyroid symptoms and risk factors. And if your doctor refuses even to test for a thyroid problem, my best advice is to look for a new doctor.

HELP! I'VE BEEN DIAGNOSED AND I *STILL* CAN'T LOSE WEIGHT!

I hear from so many people who gained weight before being diagnosed with hypothyroidism. Their doctors sometimes suggest that the weight gained while becoming hypothyroid will be lost after starting on the thyroid hormone replacement. Some people even think it will automatically melt off.

This does happen for *some* people . . . but not for everyone, and not even for the majority. It certainly didn't happen for me, and for hundreds of people who write to me each month complaining about just this problem or the thousands of posts to my bulletin board that bemoan difficulties losing weight.

You might assume your metabolism will return to normal once you're on thyroid hormone replacement. The doctor might have told you that after the magic "two weeks"—or for some doctors "six weeks"—after starting thyroid hormone replacement your system would return to normal. You may interpret this to mean that you will be able to maintain your weight while eating and exercising as you did before you had a thyroid problem. Or you might assume you could lose weight in the same way as you did before becoming hypothyroid.

Again, this does happen for *some* people. But probably not for the majority, despite what doctors say.

Katie, a marathon runner with hypothyroidism, was desperate to lose weight. She told her doctor that she was eating a healthy diet of 1,200 calories a day and jogging five miles daily. Her doctor's response? "Get off the couch and stop eating so much!"

It's mystifying, frankly. If weight gain is listed in the medical textbooks as a symptom that should trigger an examination for hypothyroidism, why does it mysteriously become an unrelated issue the minute after you fill a prescription?

What I'm suggesting is that you shouldn't expect much in the way of sympathy from the conventional doctors and endocrinologists when it comes to difficulty losing weight. Other patients can sympathize. I can definitely sympathize. But don't be disappointed if your doctor gives you a "get off the couch" or "eat less" response. Once you're diagnosed and in the normal TSH range, most of them simply don't believe your thyroid has much to do with weight issues.

Don't look to the patient groups to have a handle on this issue either. A Thyroid Foundation of America brochure says:

> Now we know that if your thyroid begins to make too little hormone, you may slow down and take less exercise—but you won't gain a lot of weight just because of having less hormone.

The thyroid is a master gland of metabolism. Think of metabolism as the engine in a standard transmission car. The car can idle at 2,000 RPM and burn a small amount of fuel each minute. Or it can idle at 4,000 RPM and burn larger amounts of fuel per minute.

When your metabolism isn't functioning well, you're idling slow, burning less. You may not be as energetic as usual, so you get less exercise, have less spring in your step, generally move less, which lowers your caloric requirements. Even if you eat the same amount as you might have eaten a few short months before, you might gain weight, or find it difficult to lose without cutting back even more calories than usual.

But as I mentioned, some people with hypothyroidism—even athletes—are moving as fast and as much as always, and still find it incredibly difficult to lose or maintain their normal weight. Insufficient exercise and activity is not reason enough to explain their weight problems. I theorize that many people with hypothyroidism are up against three different factors that have an impact on our ability to lose weight:

- a changed metabolic "set point"
- changes in brain chemistry due to illness and stress
- insulin resistance

METABOLIC SET POINT

According to Dr. Lou Aronne, author of the bestselling book *Weigh Less Live Longer*, when you begin to take in too many calories, you can gain a small amount of weight. Your body recognizes the starting weight as your "set point." Then, in order to maintain your set point weight: "your metabolism speeds up to process the excess calories, your appetite decreases, and some of the newly gained weight drops off."

According to Dr. Aronne, this self-regulating process is known as metabolic resistance.

Dr. Aronne and other weight-loss experts believe that just as your body works to maintain a temperature "set point" of 98.6, it also appears to work toward maintaining a particular weight. His theory is that, in people with a chronic weight problem, the body puts up only modest metabolic resistance to weight gain. If you continue to take in more calories than you burn, the metabolic resistance loses strength, and your body then establishes a new, higher weight set point.

What this means is, if several years ago, a woman at five feet, seven inches and 160 pounds needed 2,500 calories a day to maintain her weight, and now, after a diagnosis of hypothyroidism and a steady weight gain, at 210 pounds, she needs 2,800 calories to maintain her weight, if she dropped her calories back to 2,500, would she lose the extra 50 pounds? No. Because as she reduces her calories and loses weight, her metabolic rate slows down. According to Dr. Aronne, she would probably drop to about 197 pounds, although she'd be consuming the same number of calories as another woman of the same height who's stayed steady at 160 pounds.

My theory is that because the body is in a state of hypometabolism—underfunctioning metabolism—in hypothyroidism, the metabolic resistance becomes impaired, allowing the body to establish more easily a higher set point, and making it harder to lose weight.

CHANGES IN BRAIN CHEMISTRY

Hunger is intricately tied to brain chemistry. According to Dr. Aronne, the hypothalamus in your brain senses you need energy and issues a brain chemical with the message "eat carbohydrates." That brain chemical surge is what you feel as "hunger." Once the hypothalamus senses you've eaten enough carbohydrates, it releases serotonin to tell the body, "okay, enough carbohydrates." Serotonin is a neurotransmitter involved not only in appetite, but depression, mood, and sleep.

This system can be dramatically altered by a process present in chronic thyroid disease:

- thyroid disease slows down the metabolism.
- your metabolism is then too slow for the appetite level set by your brain.
- what your brain perceives as appropriate food intake levels then exceed your body's metabolism, creating weight gain.

When you have chronic hypothyroidism, your body is under stress, which interferes with the brain chemistry and can reduce the release of serotonin. In fact, part of the weight-loss success of the recalled diet drugs "Fen-Phen" (fenfluramine phenteremine) for some people with hypothyroidism was the fact that they increased serotonin and created a feeling of satisfaction and fullness.

INSULIN RESISTANCE

Insulin is a hormone released by the pancreas. When you eat foods that contain carbohydrates (which make up the majority of most of our diets), your body converts the carbohydrates into simple sugars. These sugars enter the blood, becoming "blood sugar." Your pancreas then releases insulin to stimulate the cells to take in the blood sugar and store it as an energy reserve, returning blood sugar levels to normal.

Carbohydrates can be "simple," high-glycemic (high-sugar) carbohydrates such as pasta, bread, sugar, white flour, and cakes, or "complex," lower-glycemic (lower-sugar), higher-fiber carbohydrates, like fruits, vegetables, and whole grains. This is an important point some people miss: fruits and vegetables are *carbohydrates*.

Some scientists speculate that sugars and starches are more easily broken down today than in our prehistoric past. They claim that many of us do not need and cannot process the amounts of carbohydrates that are considered "normal" by current dietary standards. Some scientists speculate that for as much as 25 percent of the population, eating what appears to be a "normal amount" of carbohydrates may, in fact, raise blood sugar to excessive levels. The pancreas responds by increasing the secretion of insulin to a level where it will drive down blood sugar. For this group, consistently eating too many carbohydrates—and remember that what is too many for this group is not necessarily too many for the average person—creates a situation called "insulin resistance."

Insulin resistance means that cells have become less responsive to the effects of insulin. So your body has to produce more and more insulin in order to maintain normal blood sugar levels. The insulin can also remain in your blood in higher concentrations. This is known as hyperinsulinemia.

In addition to those who seem to have a lowered need for carbohydrates, some people simply eat too many carbohydrates. Today's low-fat diets emphasize more and more pasta, bagels, and sugary fat-free products, and most of these are high-glycemic carbohydrates. There's some evidence that basic overconsumption of high-glycemic foods can trigger insulin resistance and weight gain.

If you are insulin-resistant, eating carbohydrates can make you crave more carbohydrates. You'll gain weight more easily and have difficulty losing it. There are some estimates that 25 percent of the general population, and 75 percent of overweight people, are insulin-resistant.

High insulin levels can stimulate your appetite, making you feel hungrier than normal for carbohydrate-rich food, while lowering the amount of sugar your body burns as energy and making your cells more effective at storing fat, less able to remove fat.

When you're creating this excess insulin, it also prevents your body from using its stored fat for energy. Hence, your insulin response to excess carbohydrates causes you to gain weight, or you cannot lose weight. Weight problems are not the worst aspect of insulin resistance. Insulin resistance may set up a whole syndrome of other serious health problems, including diabetes, increased risk of coronary artery disease, high blood pressure, and high cholesterol.

It makes sense that hypothyroidism, with its penchant for slowing down everything else in our systems right down to our cells, can also slow down our body's ability to process carbohydrates and our cells' ability to absorb blood sugar. The carbohydrates we could once eat, then become too much to handle. Excess carbohydrates equals excess insulin equals excess weight. And that excess weight is a double whammy because hypothyroidism already increases the risk of high cholesterol, heart disease, and diabetes.

Interestingly, many of the unrelieved symptoms we assume are also due to hypothyroidism—tiredness, dizziness, fatigue, exhaustion, uncontrolled hunger—may, in fact, be side effects of blood sugar swings due to insulin resistance. Any illness, such as the chronic thyroid problems we all face, also creates physical stress. And stress raises cortisol levels. And overproduction of cortisol increases insulin levels.

All these factors mean that insulin resistance is probably even more of a factor for overweight people with hypothyroidism than for the general population.

If you've tried conventional low-fat diets that are heavy on fruits, vegetables, pasta, rice, and grains, and low on protein and good fats, and find that you can't lose weight, or even gain weight, you might be insulin-resistant.

HOW TO LOSE WEIGHT WITH HYPOTHYROIDISM

When you look at the issue of metabolic set point, changes in brain chemistry due to illness and stress, and insulin resistance, compounded by the underlying fatigue and lack of energy that can accompany hypothyroidism, it may seem nearly impossible to get weight under control. But it's not impossible!

There are specific things that may help. Many of the people with hypothyroidism who have successfully lost weight, after battling it in other ways, have done so via a combination of the following methods.

Antidepressants or Supplements

Even if you do not suffer from depression, you might find that you have greater success fighting a stubborn weight problem if your doctor tries you on a course of antidepressants. A number of people have written to report that their diet/exercise plan suddenly began to work after their doctor prescribed a short course of antidepressant medication, like Prozac, Welbutrin, or Paxil, for example. It's worth discussing with your doctor.

Some antidepressants have side effects, and in some cases, people simply prefer natural supplements. Alternative medicine expert Andrew Weil, M.D., recommends the herbal treatment called St. John's Wort (*Hypericum perforatum*), which has components that are similar to tricyclic depressants. If you take St. John's Wort, be sure that you are getting an extremely reliable brand name, as extreme variations in potency have been found. Personally, I've found St. John's Wort to be much more effective for me, surprisingly, than prescription drugs.

Others have had success with a supplement called 5 HTP, 5-Hydroxytryptophan, an amino acid derivative and the immediate precursor to serotonin. This is one I say approach with caution. The only people I know who have tried this, myself included, have had energy "crashes" on this. I don't know if our experiences are unusual, but it's worth a warning.

Regular Aerobic Exercise

As a confirmed couch potato whose major athletic feats are yoga and walking, I'm the last person to talk about exercise. But there's no doubt that exercise is as potent a medicine as you can get and appears to be one of the factors that is absolutely *essential* to healthy weight loss or weight maintenance with hypothyroidism.

First, regular aerobic exercise is a completely natural way to help the serotonin problem. Dr. Weil recommends at least 30 minutes of some vigorous aerobic activity at least five times a week as a natural mood elevator and antidepressant.

Second, exercise—both aerobic and muscle-building exercises such as weight training—raises metabolism and can offset some of the metabolic slowdown that seems to plague even those of us with treated hypothyroidism.

Third, according to Jean-Pierre Despres, Ph.D., Professor of Medicine and Physical Education and Director of the Lipid Research Center at Laval University Hospital in Quebec:

> Exercise is probably the best medication on the market to treat insulin resistance syndrome. . . . Our studies show that low-intensity, prolonged exercise—such as a daily brisk walk of forty-five minutes to an hour—will substantially reduce insulin levels.

Geri, a health writer and television producer in New York, says keeping her weight stable requires exercise:

Exercise makes a *huge* difference. Even when I was at my most exhausted, I dragged my butt out of bed and did a little low-intensity exercise about five mornings a week. My schedule now is pretty crazy and I work long hours, so I don't have tons of time to exercise, but I do about twenty to thirty minutes of aerobics or light weight training about five days a week. Nothing major, but so far it seems to do the trick. When I slip off this habit a little, I find that I get more tired and slightly "hypo feeling"—sluggish, easily distracted, weak.

Okay, it's clear that we all need to get moving!! But that's not always very easy. Some people say, "But I'm hypothyroid, I'm exhausted all the time, and now you're telling me to exercise on top of it all?" The answer is: YES! But sometimes you have to start very slowly.

Cynthia White, a certified aerobic instructor and personal trainer from Denton, Texas, herself has hypothyroidism. With her perspective, she has some excellent advice regarding exercise and working activity into your life:

First of all, start small. Set goals that you can accomplish. It is much more motivating to continue on any new habit if you achieve small victories along the way.

So many people with hypothyroidism fight fatigue, which makes them less energetic and motivated to exercise. According to Cynthia, there are ways to offset this:

Figure out when your peak energy period is. For some people it is in the morning, other people get their energy at night. Pinpoint your peak and do something active at that time. You also have to mentally motivate yourself. What is more motivating? Your appearance or your health? If it is your appearance, go through fitness magazines and cut out pictures of people that motivate you. (I used to paste them up on my refrigerator!) If it's your health, list all the benefits of exercise. There are too many to list here but a sampling includes a lower risk for breast cancer, improved cardiovascular system, increased energy, increased self-esteem, and the list could go on.

If you don't enjoy working out, the trick, according to Cynthia, is to find something you enjoy doing . . . walking, tennis, racquetball, or swimming. She suggests you find an activity that you and your spouse or friend could do together, like take a walk, and think of it as precious time to talk to each other.

Cynthia also suggests weight lifting:

Muscle is more metabolically active than fat. You don't even have to go to a gym to do this. Just buy a couple of sets of dumbbells, one set in five pounds and one in ten pounds, and do the routine at home. Setting up a "circuit type" routine will kill two birds with one stone. You will be working aerobically and lifting at the same time. One myth-buster: unless you are genetically blessed with a mesomorph body type (one that has a tendency to add muscle easily, which is rare for women) you will not "bulk up!" Trust me, I have been lifting for years and haven't bulked up yet. There are many books that can set you up with a basic weight training program. The idea is to work the muscles like your legs, back, chest, arms, and shoulders.

Cynthia also emphasizes that there are a multitude of ways to incorporate activity into the everyday tasks of life:

Take the stairs, park farther out in the parking lot. Get up off the couch and turn the channel on the TV. Don't go through the drive-through; get out of your car and go into the store. If you work in an office, find reasons to get up out of your chair. When you are sitting, wiggle or tap your foot. It may be small, but it requires energy.

Finally, Cynthia recommends that to stick to your new habit, start by setting a reasonable goal:

You will be surprised at how good you will feel from exercising, achieving your goal, and reaping benefits such as increased energy! If you can stick with even small changes, they will lead to small successes, and you will create a snowball effect, rolling your way into healthy and fun lifestyle changes. Take the plunge!

It seems that people with hypothyroidism *need* exercise about as much as we need our thyroid hormone pills. Even if you're not a health spa or gym sort of person, the health experts tout the basic benefits of walking. Even a few minutes of brisk walking every day would be more exercise than the majority of us ever gets and a terrific goal to accomplish. So consider this a hypothyroidism prescription for a lifetime: Rx—take a walk and get moving!!

Breathing

It goes by a variety of names. In yoga, it's pranayama, the art and science of breathing. In marketing language it's Breathercise or Oxycise. Some of the diet centers are even incorporating it into their programs. Whatever you call it, a program of deep breathing exercises, designed to take in more oxygen and release more carbon dioxide with each breath, seems to help many people with hypothyroidism to lose weight.

We know that hypothyroidism affects the strength of your respiratory muscles. Hypothyroidism is also known to increase reactivity of the bronchial passages, even if you don't have asthma. Even when treated, a substantial percentage of people with hypothyroidism report "shortness of breath," "feeling like they're not getting enough oxygen," or even "needing to yawn to get more air" as continuing symptoms.

For many of us, the ability to take in and process oxygen may be forever changed once hypothyroidism sets in. Even when fully treated, I suspect that most of us still don't take in and process oxygen fully. That is why specific attention to breathing seems to help some people with hypothyroidism.

Most doctors will probably tell you that this is a load of hooey. You want to lose weight, "get off the couch and stop eating so much!" But breathing programs seem to be working for many people who are writing to me. And, unless you actually ante up and pay for an Oxycise program, learning how to breathe is about as inexpensive as it can be. All you need is some air and a pair of lungs to start. And no one can say that learning to breathe better isn't good for you, thyroid problem or not.

Breathing experts point to numerous health benefits of systematic breathing practice, including:

- increases oxygen delivery to the cells, which helps provide sufficient energy to fuel metabolism
- aids in weight loss and digestion
- reduces fatigue, increases energy
- reduces stress, allows for greater relaxation and inner peace

If you're interested in trying out better breathing for yourself, you can start by learning deep abdominal breathing. Here's a simple breathing exercise to try:

> Lie on your back, body relaxed. Put your hand on your abdomen. Take a deep, slow breath through your nose, filling your belly, so your hand rises. Then exhale slowly, letting all the air out of your belly. Inhale again, filling the abdomen until your hand rises. Again, exhale. Feel the breath energy rising from the abdomen to the throat, and back down again to the abdomen.

You can start practicing this deep, abdominal breathing anywhere. Sitting in the car, standing in line, in the shower. It's a first step toward incorporating deep breathing into your daily life. Several times a day, stop and just focus on your breathing. Take a few deep abdominal breaths. Every time you feel tired, try taking five deep abdominal breaths. See if these ventures in breathing practice help you feel even a bit more energetic or alert.

If you want to delve into breathing to help your metabolism, I strongly recommend a wonderful book that has everything you need to know about breathing for metabolism, Pam Grout's *Jumpstart Your Metabolism*. Pam became a breathing coach after she successfully lost weight by learning special metabolism-oriented breathing techniques. Pam goes through a variety of different breathing exercises you can do to help increase metabolism. In addition to learning yoga breathing exercises in yoga class, Pam's book is where I've learned the best techniques to improve my own breathing.

A Low-Glycemic Diet

An effective method to combat insulin resistance and the inability to properly process simple carbohydrates is eating a low-glycemic, low-fat diet. Low-glycemic foods are foods that do not rank high on the "glycemic index," a ranking that assigns values to foods based on their effect on your blood sugar.

High-glycemic foods are sugary, starchy foods like pasta, rice, white flour breads, cereal, desserts, and sugary drinks. You may feel frustrated that there's nothing left to eat. But you need to rethink your eating habits, shifting to a diet of low-fat protein sources (like beans, legumes, chicken, turkey, fish, lean red meat) and nonstarchy vegetables and fruits, and certain grains.

If you have Internet access, the gold standard for information on the low-glycemic diet is featured at Rick Mendosa's "Glycemic Index" page, at *http://www.cruzio.com/~mendosa/gi.htm*. Rick has comprehensive charts outlining the glycemic values of various foods, as well as excellent links to the other Web sites and the latest information on glycemic values.

The book I found most useful is *Dr. Bob Arnot's Revolutionary Weight Control Program* by the NBC "Today" show's resident medical advisor, Doctor Bob Arnot. In addition to including excellent charts on the glycemic values of different foods, Dr. Bob's book encourages eating what he refers to as "hard" foods versus "soft" foods. Hard foods are higher-fiber foods that require more energy to process and digest, and thus burn more calories. Other helpful books are discussed in the Resources appendix.

WHAT IF THIS DOESN'T WORK?

Dana Laake, MS, RDH, LN, a well-respected preventive and therapeutic nutritionist, speaking at a women's health conference in 1998, was asked a question about the diets that were popular at the time. These included "Sugar Busters," which is a form of a low-glycemic diet, the Atkins Diet, and Barry Sears' popular Zone diet. These diets have been criticized by conventional doctors as "radical," too "high-protein," not low-fat enough for weight loss or not balanced enough. Dana gave what I thought was excellent advice:

> No one diet is necessarily right for you. But if you're not losing weight eating the way you're eating now, change the way you're eating. You can try one of these diets, and see if it has an effect. Then, starting there, you can work your way back toward a healthier, balanced version of that diet.

This is excellent advice, recognizing that any one diet is not the answer for everyone. Conventional low-fat diets will help some hypothyroid people lose weight. High-fiber diets may be the key for others.

The point is to take a look at whatever way of eating you're following now, and if it isn't working, try something very different, perhaps even radical, and see if that has an effect. Once you determine that a vegetarian, low-glycemic, high-fiber, Zone, or other diet might be effective, you can experiment to find a healthy, balanced version of that diet that works best for you.

CHAPTER 10

Depression and
Hypothyroidism

*Believe, when you are most unhappy, that there is something for
you to do in the world.*
HELEN KELLER

The relationship between hypothyroidism and depression is, first, very real and, second, somewhat complicated. There are three key ways hypothyroidism and depression are related.

First, chapter 3 discussed how depression is a common symptom of hypothyroidism. Second, a diagnosis of depression may actually be a misdiagnosis that overlooks the real problem: hypothyroidism. And, third, depression can persist in people with hypothyroidism, even when the thyroid problem has been treated. Let's take a look at these issues.

DEPRESSION—A MISDIAGNOSIS OF HYPOTHYROIDISM

Depression is very common in the United States. According to the National Institute of Mental Health, depression affects approximately 17.6 million Americans each year. It is estimated that 5 to 12 percent of men and 10 to 20 percent of women in the U.S. will suffer from a major depressive episode at some time in their life. Some researchers estimate that as many as 25 million people in the United States take antidepressants to treat major depression and the less severe form of depression known as "dysthymia" (diss-THY-me-ah).

Depression is more common than hypothyroidism, which affects an estimated 13 million Americans. Some of the symptoms of depression are also quite similar to those of hypothyroidism, including a depressed, sad and/or anxious mood, difficulty concentrating, sleeping difficulties, fatigue, loss of energy, change in weight, and irritability. Also similar is the fact that depression is more common in women: in fact, major depression and dysthymia affect twice as many women as men.

Because, statistically, symptoms are more likely to be coming from depression than hypothyroidism, many doctors will offer a diagnosis of depression without testing for thyroid disease. Some doctors and managed care systems also tend to avoid the added expense of thyroid testing when depression is the primary symptom.

Peg's doctors were so convinced that her health problems were due to depression that she spent five years in therapy trying to get rid of her symptoms before being diagnosed and treated for hypothyroidism.

> It's funny in a way that I allowed the voice of a doctor (or anyone else for that matter) to overpower my own . . . to make me doubt what my body has been telling me, *loudly,* for five years. I don't regret all the therapy I've sought out, trying in vain to get to the core of why I "made myself sick." But this *wasn't* in my head, and so no matter how hard I tried, it wouldn't go away.

It's clear that many doctors just don't think of hypothyroidism when faced with a patient complaining of depression, *even when other hypothyroidism symptoms are present.* So there's a definite risk of misdiagnosis.

Studies have even shown that, among patients hospitalized for depression, 15 percent of them have previously undiagnosed subclinical hypothyroidism. Tom was one of those patients. When he first started getting sick, his doctor labeled him as depressed and prescribed Prozac and Xanax. Tom ended up hospitalized for depression, until a tenacious doctor decided to test his thyroid, and discovered that his symptoms—mood swings, eating problems, sleep problems, weight gain, and depression—were due to serious hypothyroidism.

Mike, whose wife Sherry was newly diagnosed with hypothyroidism, found out firsthand how easily doctors attribute medical problems to depression:

> They could not find any medical reason for my wife's problems, so they blamed it on psychosis. The doctor said "you need for her to see a psychiatrist." Some of her complaints were weakness, confusion, loss of appetite, frequent bladder infections, and too many other complaints to mention. I know my wife, and I knew that she was not mentally ill. I ended up taking her home after she started on the thyroid hormone, and each day I could see improvement in her condition.

Several research studies have concluded that thyroid-function screening should be required for all patients with depression, psychosis, or organic mental disorder. Instead of ending up in mental health facilities, or on antidepressant therapy that doesn't work, patients would be tested at the onset, and many could avoid months or years of inappropriate and ineffective treatment for the wrong condition. Many doctors, however, still don't routinely test for a thyroid problem when a patient first complains of depression. Why they don't is a question that I think deserves to be answered by the medical profession.

Unfortunately, when hypothyroidism is the actual cause of depression, and a person has been misdiagnosed as depressed, prescribed antidepressants may help slightly but aren't likely to resolve the symptoms. The Thyroid Society estimates that 10 to 15 percent of the patients with a diagnosis of depression may have an underlying thyroid hormone deficiency. But this number may actually be higher, especially if you consider that high-normal TSH values may in fact reflect subclinical hypothyroidism for some people.

Some researchers have reported that 80 percent of the estimated 25 million people in the United States who take antidepressants still suffer a variety of unresolved symptoms—particularly weight gain, lethargy, and loss of libido. Interestingly, these are also the very same symptoms of hypothyroidism. How many of these people are misdiagnosed and are actually suffering from hypothyroidism? It's a good question that also deserves to be answered by the medical establishment.

Christine, a woman with hypothyroidism who suffered from depression before her diagnosis, recommends that you listen to your instincts: "I probably would have committed myself to a mental institution by now if I didn't know in my heart that my depression was due to my thyroid."

While we wait for answers, in the meantime, if you or someone you know has been diagnosed with depression, insist on having a thyroid test right from the start. The good news is that, in most cases, depression and psychiatric problems caused by hypothyroidism will lessen and eventually go away with sufficient thyroid hormone replacement therapy.

PERSISTENT DEPRESSION WITH HYPOTHYROIDISM

There is no doubt that having hypothyroidism is a key risk factor for depression. According to the Thyroid Society for Education and Research, most patients with hypothyroidism have some degree of associated depression, ranging from mild to severe. Ron Pies, M.D., a clinical professor of psychiatry at Tufts University and *Psychiatric Times* columnist, estimated that as many as 40 percent of clinically hypothyroid patients have significant depression.

Dr. Pies has speculated that there may be three reasons for the link between hypothyroidism and depression. First, a malfunctioning thyroid may actually be a marker for depression. Second, having a thyroid problem may make it easier to develop depression, or worsen the symptoms of depression. And third, depression may somehow make it easier to develop autoimmune thyroid problems leading to hypothyroidism.

Whatever the causes, for many people, the depression associated with hypothyroidism is partially or fully relieved with sufficient thyroid hormone treatment. However, even after treatment for hypothyroidism, the depression can continue in some cases. This continued depression may be a coincidence, unrelated to the hypothyroidism, it may be the body's reaction to chronic illness, or it may be an indicator that the hypothyroidism is being under-treated, or not treated correctly.

If all your other hypothyroidism symptoms have been relieved by the thyroid hormone replacement, and only depression remains, then it is worthwhile to discuss treatment for depression with your doctor. However, if you still suffer depression along with continued hypothyroidism symptoms, before accepting a diagnosis of depression, you may want to be extra diligent to ensure that you are receiving optimal treatment for your underlying thyroid problem. That may involve a dosage change, a change in brand, or specifically, the addition of T3 drugs.

I'm not saying not to pursue treatment for depression when it's needed. But make sure your thyroid problem is being treated as much as possible before letting a doctor tell you that your continued symptoms are due to depression.

Doctors in the psychopharmacological community, unlike their colleagues in endocrinology, seem to be in tune with the concerns about undertreatment in the face of normal TSH values, and the need, in some cases, for T3 drugs to help relieve depression in hypothyroid patients. This is evident, for example, in a lengthy exchange posted online at "Dr. Bob's Psychopharmacology Tips," a compilation of tips and exchanges created by Robert Hsiung, M.D., an Assistant Professor of Clinical Psychiatry at the University of Chicago.

One doctor mentions that he feels hypothyroid patients on thyroid replacement therapy need to have their TSH in the lowest quarter of the normal range (that's in the .5 to 1.75 TSH level in a normal range of .5 to 5.5) in order to respond to antidepressants. He says that getting these patients the levels of medication they need can, in some cases, be difficult, as endocrinologists seem to target levels at the top of the normal range. Another doctor indicated that he resorted to running TRH stimulation tests in order to prove continued hypothyroidism to endocrinologists or internists who objected to increases in patients' dosages. The TRH tests nearly always showed that they were on inadequate replacement therapy.

OTHER HELP FOR DEPRESSION

If your depression is a separate, coincidental issue, or is unrelieved by even you and your doctor's best efforts at treating underlying hypothyroidism, then the depression itself may also need to be treated. This is not something to be embarrassed about and doesn't reflect on your mental state. It's just an indication that your brain chemistry is interrelated with your endocrine system, and without balance in one, it's hard to get perfect balance in the other. Antidepressant treatments—such as conventional medications, herbal drugs, therapy, exercise, and support—can help balance that brain chemistry and relieve the depression.

Antidepressant Medication

The conventional treatment is antidepressant medication. Medications include some of the newer drugs, such as mirtazapine (Remeron), venlafaxine (Effexor) nefazodone (Serzone), and bupropion (Wellbutrin); the selective serotonin reuptake inhibitors (SSRIs) such as paroxetine (Paxil), fluoxetine (Prozac), and sertraline (Zoloft); the monoamine oxidase inhibitors (MAOIs) such as phenelzine (Nardil) and tranylcypromine (Parnate); and the older tricyclic antidepressants such as sinequan (Adapin), amitriptyline (Elavil), desipramine (Norpramin), imipramine (Tofranil); and others. Your doctor will need to discuss the best option for you. Remember that if you take an antidepressant, it can take a few weeks, or even as much as a month or two, to start seeing the benefits. Don't give up after a week or two if you don't notice a difference. Also, keep in mind that some antidepressants can become stronger or weaker in the presence of thyroid hormone, or can interfere with your thyroid hormone absorption, so discuss this with your doctor.

Even after starting thyroid hormone replacement, Terri continued to suffer various mental side effects from her hypothyroidism:

> My endocrinologist did not see mental side effects as valid. I thought I was losing my mind. The only way I've managed to survive this ordeal mentally is thanks to my general practitioner, who recognized my mental state. He advised that I should take an antidepressant until

my thyroid becomes completely normal. This was my lifeline. My endocrinologist never suggested this, never discussed mental side affects, and even brushed off questions I asked about them as not being scientifically proven. Thanks to the combination of treatments, especially the antidepressant, I am able to cope with the mental affects of thyroid disease.

Alternative Antidepressant Supplements

Since there are side effects associated with many antidepressants, some people try supplements. Many people try the herbal treatment St. John's Wort (hypericum perforatum). Research has found the herbal antidepressant effective in treating mild to moderately severe depression. A reminder: make sure you get an extremely reliable brand name of St. John's Wort, as some less responsible companies have been known to market extremely sub-potent St. John's Wort. A common dosage is 300 mg. of St. John's Wort, three times per day, for a total of 900 mg. Other supplements used for depression include 5 HTP, 5-Hydroxytryptophan, an amino acid derivative and the immediate precursor to serotonin, a brain chemical responible for feelings of well-being. Another supplement some find effective is tyrosine, an amino acid that is used to create norepinephrine. Norepinephrine is a brain chemical that works as an appetite suppressant, stimulant and antidepressant, and many leading-edge researchers are proposing that depression stems directly from a deficiency of norepinephrine. Again, most people need to take these supplements for at least two to three weeks in order to begin seeing some definite benefits.

A piece of advice: self-treating depression with supplements isn't a good idea. If you want to experiment with St. John's Wort, 5HTP, tyrosine or other supplements, it's a good idea to do it under the guidance of a health practitioner.

Therapy

Traditional treatment for mild and moderate cases of depression can also include psychotherapy. Counseling or therapy—even short-term—can be useful in coping with depression, particularly in learning how to prevent and deal with various sources of stress in your life, and how to cope with that stress effectively. Therapy may not cure your thyroid, but emotional stress has a tremendous impact on disease. Learning and mastering skills to cope with stress helps to ensure that the stress has the least amount of impact on your health.

Bobbi found that seeing a therapist helped her tremendously.

> I was a very negative, stressed out, worried person before, who was always an overachiever. I was experiencing some depression due to my health problems and my inability to work for over a year. I'm learning not to worry so much, and to let go of things. It has helped my health.

Exercise

Many doctors believe that aerobic exercise is the best, natural anti-depressant, and recommend 30 minutes of vigorous aerobics at least five times a week. Others have found that simply brisk walking twenty to thirty minutes daily can have a strong antidepressant effect. However you look at it, though, exercise stimulates a variety of positive things in the brain chemistry that can help to counteract depression and is therefore an essential treatment in almost every antidepressant program.

Support and Empowerment

Sue, who is a regular participant in and trained patient facilitator for depression support group meetings has many excellent suggestions for those who, like her, battle depression:

> Depression can creep up on you, sometimes without your even realizing it (although it's no one's fault). Some things (in addition to antidepressant and thyroid medication) that helped me to turn my thinking back to positive (and which I continue to use) were:
>
> • Treating myself to long soaking baths, complete with candles and nice music—in the middle of the day.

- Taking short walks. This I had to absolutely force myself to do, but cannot argue with the results; I always felt better afterward.
- Giving myself permission not to answer the phone or door if I didn't feel like it.
- Joining a support group for depression, just for women, sponsored by the Mental Health Association. Check your area, if interested.
- Being sure to get my nutrition via supplements if I wasn't eating right (too many comfort foods!).
- Going into therapy—with someone who specialized in depression—to work through my "issues." I really believe this is helpful for the future, too. If more issues are resolved, then there should be fewer things to dwell upon (negatively) in the future, in case the chemistry begins to go south (depression).
- Trying to alternate my isolation with times of sharing how I felt with friends and family.
- Trying positive self-talk—it works! Bought a book by Louise Hay, and there is really something to this ability we have of breaking cyclical negative thinking with positive reinforcement. You can use the tiniest thing you like about yourself to your extreme advantage by reminding yourself of it . . . repeatedly. Do you like your eyes? Your hair? Your compassion? Anything! The best part is you don't even have to believe that it works for it to work.
- Staying in constant touch with my family physician, in case there's a possible physical cause of the depression. Such was the case with my thyroid problem. Oh, I don't believe it was the total cause, but definitely a contribution. The depression can cause us to forget about this aspect of our health. And when it comes to thyroid problems, they're not always revealed with standard testing.
- Getting an advocate for myself, to deal with the endless paperwork, telephone contacts (i.e., insurance), and other details. In my case, it was my sister, but there are organizations offering this as a free service to the disabled.

Finally, many people like Sue find that giving and receiving support is of tremendous value in dealing with their depression. Consider getting involved in a local support group for depression, where you can exchange support and information with others.

CHAPTER 11

Infertility, Pregnancy, and Hypothyroidism

Of all the rights of women, the greatest is to be a mother.
LIN YÜ-TANG

I take a particular interest in the issues of fertility and pregnancy because I was diagnosed with Hashimoto's thyroiditis six months after I got married. Two years later, my husband and I decided we'd try to have a baby. At the time, I was thirty-four, and though I was being treated for my thyroid problem, I was still dealing with symptoms of hypothyroidism. I figured if there was a candidate for a fertility problem, it was me. So I read relentlessly, talked to a number of doctors, and tried to find out exactly how I could, first, maximize my chance of getting pregnant, and, second, ensure a healthy pregnancy.

To be honest, underlying it all was my concern that I'd need to prove that we'd specifically tried to get pregnant and had documented all the cycles and such. That way, I wouldn't have to go through the requisite year of trying to get pregnant, only to be told to start charting temperatures and testing for ovulation for another six months before I could *finally* be labeled "infertile" and start investigating fertility treatments.

I started with the books on thyroid disease. Unfortunately, most of the patient-oriented literature was not much help. The books mentioned that untreated hypothyroidism increases the risk of infertility, miscarriage, or complications, but that once treated, these issues would no longer be a problem. End of discussion.

For a disease that affects mainly women, this glossing over of the diseases' effect on reproduction—a very important time for a women healthwise—seems irresponsible, indicative of how little the medical profession seems to understand the impact hypothyroidism has on a woman's ability to live well and live normally.

With little information available, I was determined to research the issue myself to make sure that I had the best possible outcome. First, I needed to make sure that all the reproductive basics were covered, meaning I needed to answer a key question: Was I ovulating and when?

Hypothyroidism, especially untreated, but also when *under*-treated, can cause anovulation, the fancy term for not ovulating. When you don't ovulate, there's no egg to fertilize, so conception becomes impossible, hence, no pregnancy. You may still have periods, however, so don't assume you're ovulating or ovulating regularly if you still have periods. Hypothyroidism can also cause irregular ovulation, which can result in menstrual irregularities and cycle changes. For example, after twenty years of periods every 28 days like clockwork, once hypothyroid, my periods came every 23-26 days, irregularly.

Another fertility concern related to hypothyroidism is what's known as a short luteal phase. The luteal phase is the time between when you ovulate and when your period begins. A normal luteal phase is approximately thirteen to fifteen days. The luteal phase needs to be long enough to nurture a fertilized egg. Too short a luteal phase can cause what appears to be infertility but is, in fact, failure to sustain a fertilized egg, with loss of the very early pregnancy at about the same time that your period would typically begin.

I started by charting my basal body temperatures in order to monitor fertility signs and ovulation, and determine my luteal phase. My bible was a book that is, in my opinion, absolutely essential for all women, called *Taking Charge of Your Fertility*, by Toni Wechsler, MPH. With this book, I learned (for the first time I might add) the real story about the menstrual and hormonal cycles. This book is definitely a far cry from those *Now You're a Woman* pamphlets and films in grade school. I learned how to use basal temperature and other fertility signs to chart my monthly hormonal cycle. While charting allowed me to estimate ovulation, I also used an over-the-counter ovulation predictor kit, available for around $10 at the drugstore, to confirm ovulation, to make sure I knew what I was doing with the charting. After three months, according to my charts and testing, it was obvious I was ovulating, and I had a long enough luteal phase to sustain pregnancy. That was a good start.

I had already scheduled a "preconception" appointment with the doctor a few months earlier, which had resulted in my getting an overdue measles/mumps/rubella vaccination and a prescription for the extra folic acid that is essential in the period prior to and during pregnancy to prevent birth defects.

In addition to the pre-pregnancy preparation I had done with my regular doctors, I also decided to consult with the endocrinologist, just to make sure things were in good shape thyroidwise. My TSH level at the time was 4.1. I was feeling okay, not perfect, but pretty well, and thought that because I was in normal range, this would be a good time to finally try to get pregnant.

Not so, said my endocrinologist. She said she had found anecdotally that the optimal range to get pregnant and maintain a pregnancy is a TSH of approximately 1 to 2. (This is at a lab where normal range is .5 to 5.5, over 5.5 is considered hypothyroid.) She said there weren't any specific journal papers to back up her own findings, but she said she'd even treated fellow physicians suffering from infertility who'd been able to get pregnant once TSH was lowered to the 1 to 2 level. She said I might be able to get pregnant at my current level but to sustain a pregnancy would be more difficult. So she upped my dosage of thyroid hormone replacement, targeting the TSH range of 1 to 2.

Interestingly, there *is* some research that backs up her opinions on normal levels during early pregnancy. There's a 1994 study in the *Journal of Clinical Endocrinology and Metabolism* that looked at pregnant women with thyroid antibodies and TSH in the normal range. The study found that women with autoimmune thyroid disease had TSH values significantly higher, though still normal, in the first trimester than in women with healthy pregnancies used as controls. The higher TSH level of the women with autoimmune thyroid disease? 1.6. The *normal* TSH level for the control group of pregnant woman without autoimmune thyroid disease? 0.9. A

TSH of .9 is a far cry from the so-called "normal" TSH levels of 3 or 4 or 5 that some doctors feel are no impediment whatsoever to getting, or staying, pregnant.

Within a month, my thyroid was down to a TSH level of 1.2. The next month, planning our timing according to our fertility charts, I actually became pregnant. The whole process, charting the cycle, getting the TSH level down, and getting pregnant, took four months. I'm not going to say this is typical or normal, but it was a pleasant surprise for us, and I think the charting process, knowing exactly when I ovulated and being sure my thyroid function was optimal were all factors in the success. By assuming that getting pregnant when hypothyroid must be a long, difficult, or nearly impossible task, it turned out to be much easier than I expected.

AUTOIMMUNE THYROID
DISEASE AND INFERTILITY

I was very lucky to be able to conceive my daughter so quickly, and with a minimum of difficulty. Unfortunately, some women with thyroid problems may find they have trouble conceiving, or may suffer recurrent miscarriage, if their doctors believe that any TSH in the normal range is sufficient to get pregnant and maintain a pregnancy. If you are hypothyroid, and your doctor is in this mindset, I'd urge you to find another doctor who will consider targeting a lower TSH level, or even adding supplemental T3 to your treatment, to ensure maximum fertility and healthy pregnancy.

A separate concern is the number of women who suffer from infertility or recurrent miscarriage due to underlying autoimmune thyroid problems but who are not even aware they have this problem.

If you or someone you know is having difficulty getting pregnant, or is suffering recurrent miscarriage, thyroid antibodies should be tested. While the patient-oriented literature overlooks this entirely, some of the more pioneering medical researchers and fertility specialists understand that the presence of antithyroid antibodies— even in the absence of an elevated TSH or symptoms of hypothyroidism—can be a factor in infertility or early miscarriage. A variety of immunological adjustments need to take place in a pregnant woman, and the existence of underlying autoimmune thyroid problems may set in motion a mechanism that results in a greater incidence of infertility, lower success rates with in vitro fertilization or more frequent miscarriage.

Many doctors do not appear to know about this link between antibodies and infertility, yet it is published in conventional research journals. The respected journal *Obstetrics and Gynecology* reported that the presence of antithyroid antibodies increases the risk of miscarriage. According to U.S. research reported in the *Journal of Clinical Endocrinology and Metabolism,* that risk of miscarriage can be twice as high for women who have antithyroid antibodies.

Researchers have also demonstrated that antithyroid antibodies can cause greater difficulty conceiving after in vitro fertilization, regardless of whether or not there are clinical symptoms of hypothyroidism. Researchers had greater success in achieving successful pregnancies when they gave low doses of Heparin (an antiblood clotting agent) and aspirin and/or intravenous immunoglobulin G (IVIG) to women who had antithyroid antibodies. Dr. Geoffrey Sher and colleagues at Pacific Fertility Centers performed this research.

Keep in mind that if you are monitoring your ovulation and cycle, and have your thyroid and TSH levels regulated, and you still don't get pregnant after the requisite six months to a year, you probably should consult with a fertility specialist for additional treatment and ideas.

Colleen was diagnosed as hypothyroid when she went to see her doctor about her inability to get pregnant:

> Through my entire time of having a "cycle" it was rarely regular. I could go for a year without my period and my previous doctor had said not to worry about it until you are ready to try to have a baby. My new doctor was very concerned about this. Through all the blood tests it was discovered that I was hypothyroid. My TSH was 15. I was put on Synthroid and am monitored every six weeks. I was still not

pregnant, even though my level was just checked at .8 and I am on Synthroid .75 mcg.

Because it may be more than her thyroid involved, Colleen ended up deciding to pursue more aggressive fertility efforts, taking Clomid and Provera to induce ovulation and a cycle and going to see a reproductive endocrinologist.

For many women, proper thyroid treatment and TSH levels, however, can raise the likelihood of a successful pregnancy. To date, five women have written me to say that after extended periods of what their doctors had diagnosed as infertility, they took this information on antibodies and TSH levels, and finally insisted that their doctors test them for thyroid disease, treat high-normal TSH levels in the presence of antibodies, and/or increase their dosage of thyroid hormone to get their levels down to the 1 to 2 TSH range. And every one of those five women is now a mother for the first time.

HYPOTHYROIDISM AND PREGNANCY

Once you become pregnant, there are important things to monitor in terms of the hypothyroidism in order to ensure that the pregnancy is a healthy one for both the baby and you. Many guidelines say that a pregnant woman with hypothyroidism should have her thyroid function checked during each trimester. In particular, it's known that the thyroid hormone dosage requirement can increase in the early part of pregnancy due to the increased estrogen levels of early pregnancy. Since many women aren't even sure that they are pregnant until four to six weeks, many women don't even get in to see their doctors—and test their thyroid function—until the first trimester is more than half over. Interestingly, if you call to schedule a first visit with an obstetrician, they often aren't that concerned about getting you in that early in the pregnancy.

In my case, I tested positive via home pregnancy test only nine days postconception. This is fairly unusual. Some women who are pregnant still don't test positive until about fourteen days postconception or later. I had a blood test to confirm the pregnancy at my regular doctor's office and knew I was officially pregnant at only three weeks, which is when I called to schedule my first obstetrician (OB) appointment. My OB—recommended by my endocrinologist as an OB familiar with thyroid disease—wanted to schedule me to come in sometime in the eighth or ninth week. I insisted on scheduling the first visit at five weeks. At that time, I also asked that they run a TSH test. Interestingly, in just the five weeks of pregnancy, my TSH had gone up to 3, from 1.2. In keeping with my endocrinologist's directions, my dosage was upped slightly, I was retested two weeks later, and my TSH returned to about 1.4.

Requiring an early adjustment to dosage during pregnancy is very common. Jennifer was diagnosed in 1989 with severe hypothyroidism, with a TSH of 298. After treatment, she was in the normal TSH range, taking Synthroid at a dosage of .175:

> During my third month of pregnancy, I was so exhausted and weak, I decided to get a TSH test. The doctor, unbelievably, was reluctant, but I pressured him. As you can guess, my TSH was 90, well out of range. I now take .2 of the Synthroid. I want people to know how much pregnancy affects the thyroid levels and that you should push to have doctors do the blood tests as soon as possible.

Lily experienced the tragedy of an early miscarriage and suspects her doctor's failure to increase her thyroid hormone dosage enough may be at the root of the problem:

> Four weeks into the pregnancy my TSH was 8.45, at six weeks it was 10.5 even though my Synthroid had been increased slightly. My reproductive endocrinologist and primary care physician are saying the thyroid was not the "cause," but I am wondering then why hypothyroidism is identified as a miscarriage risk factor. I had an ultrasound at five and a half weeks and the baby looked perfect. I had another at eight weeks and there was no heartbeat.

In my case, when I called to schedule that first appointment, the nurse told me to start taking an over-the-counter prenatal vitamin with iron right away. What the nurse didn't tell me then, or the doctor didn't mention at any point during my pregnancy, is something few obstetricians or even endocrinologists will tell you about prenatal vitamins. Iron, whether in prenatal vitamins, or as separate supplements, can interfere with proper absorption of thyroid hormone, causing you to get less thyroid hormone than you need. This is a problem anytime, but particularly of concern during pregnancy, when you want to make extra sure you get enough thyroid hormone at all times. The solution is simple. You need to take the thyroid hormone at least two to three hours apart from the prenatal vitamin or iron-containing supplement. This allows you to get full absorption of the thyroid hormone without interference from the iron.

While we're on the subject of the iron in vitamins, it's worth looking at a few other things that can interfere with proper absorption of thyroid hormone. Eating a high-fiber diet and taking antacids are two activities more common during pregnancy. Both activities, however, can have an impact on absorption of thyroid medication, and thus, affect thyroid function and levels during pregnancy. To maximize absorption and make sure the proper amount of thyroid hormone is processed, doctors recommend that you take thyroid hormone without food, on an empty stomach, at least two hours after or one hour before eating, and do not take a prenatal vitamin with iron within two to three hours of taking your thyroid hormone.

Consistency is also important. If for some reason, you can't take your pill on an empty stomach, it's better to decide to take your thyroid pill every day with food, than miss taking it or take it erratically—some days with food, some days without. You may stabilize at a slightly higher dosage than if you weren't taking your pill with food, but you'll get to the right dosage.

Some women, including Corinne, wonder if they should even continue to take their thyroid hormone during pregnancy. "I'd like to know if I should stop my thyroid hormone because I really don't want to take any drugs during pregnancy that might harm the baby."

Corinne has a dangerous misconception! *Not* to take your thyroid hormone is a danger to your health, to your pregnancy, and to your child. Thyroid hormone, in proper doses, is replacing something your body needs in order to maintain a healthy pregnancy.

Insufficient thyroid hormone in early pregnancy can increase the risk of miscarriage. Later in pregnancy, it can increase the risk of stillbirth or premature delivery. And throughout the pregnancy, having an elevated TSH level can create a substantially increased risk of negatively affecting your a child's psychological development, and can result in substantially lower I.Q. levels, reduced motor skills, and problems with attention, language, and reading throughout life. Research reported in the *New England Journal of Medicine* in 1999 demonstrated, in fact, that women with untreated underactive thyroids during pregnancy are nearly four times more likely to have children with lower I.Q. scores. Overall, the greatest danger for you and your unborn baby is to think that taking thyroid at the proper dosage of hormone is bad for your baby and discontinuing your thyroid hormone replacement. Thyroid hormone is one of the few drugs in pharmaceutical category "A" (low risk) for pregnant women. Studies in pregnant women show that when taken in the proper dosage, there are no adverse effects on the fetus.

Most people I've talked to who have autoimmune hypothyroidism say they've actually felt better while pregnant. I have to say that when pregnant I felt the best I'd been since being diagnosed as hypothyroid. Naturally, I had the typical tiredness most pregnant women experience, but it was a different feeling, not the bone-numbing fatigue and brain fog I'd had with untreated hypothyroidism, but more of a sleepiness that was relieved by naps and nighttime sleep. My allergies were near nonexistent, I didn't get a single cold, flu, or other ailment. I've heard doctors speculate that some women with autoimmune diseases have immune systems that function almost perfectly during pregnancy, and I seemed to be one of them. After the first trimester, I had my thyroid tested every two months or so, and it varied no more than a few tenths of a point, requiring no adjustment in my medication throughout the entire pregnancy. It's never been so stable before or since.

My main pregnancy concern? More weight gain that I'd have liked, and a borderline blood sugar problem that the doctor said wasn't gestational diabetes, but was close to it, late in the pregnancy. I ate very healthily—I thought—but looking back, I realize my diet was very heavy in carbohydrates and fruits. I think that hypothyroidism's tendency to give some people an exaggerated insulin response and near diabetic blood sugar levels may make some pregnant women with hypothyroidism more susceptible to border-line or full-blown gestational diabetes. If I have another baby, I will definitely follow a low-glycemic diet suitable for more strictly controlling blood sugar.

Luckily, I had a noneventful pregnancy and an easy c-section (my baby was breech) and Julia was born a healthy eight and a half pounds in late 1997.

I have one important sideline tip for hypothyroid mothers-to-be. When you go to the hospital to have your baby, pack your thyroid hormone with you in your hospital overnight bag. Other-wise, it can often be a major hassle to get them to issue you your thyroid hormone in the hospital, especially if you take anything nontraditional as I do.

After enjoying a pregnancy relatively free of thyroid fluctua-tions, it was in the postpartum period that my thyroid flared back up again. Determined to breastfeed Julia, I had coaching from La Leche league, my doula (birth attendant), and the hospital's lacta-tion consultant, and felt very prepared to nurse my daughter. Julia seemed to take to it well, but after a week, she wasn't having the requisite number of diapers or sufficient weight gain to indicate that she was getting enough milk. After trying many methods of increasing milk supply recommended by the various resources I called on, Julia continued to lose weight. At the three-week point, I finally had to go add supplemental formula for Julia. I turned to pumping to help increase my milk supply, only to discover that I was able to pump about half the typical milk supply of other moth-ers at this postpartum stage. It's clear that I had a low-milk supply, probably from the beginning.

Suspecting my thyroid was out of whack, I was tested, and they discovered that I'd become very hyperthyroid, with a TSH level of less than .05. My dosage was readjusted to return me to the TSH 1 to 2 range but this never resulted in a rebound in milk supply. It may have been too late to kickstart it, or it may be that my milk supply problem had nothing to do with the thyroid function. But my lesson here is that new mothers might want to get TSH tested a few days after delivery, so dosage modifications can be made right away. Despite the low-milk supply, I did manage to successfully pump about half of Julia's needed milk until she was six months old. I am still proud of this accomplishment, given the challenges.

My milk supply issues are apparently not uncommon for women with underlying thyroid problems. Often, a period of low-milk supply may, in fact, be a sign of postpartum thyroid problems. After suffering from a period of low-milk supply after the birth of her son, Sharon began to develop other symptoms, including sore and numb wrists and arms, and major fatigue, that she would discover were related to a case of postpartum hypothyroidism:

> I saw my internist and asked for a referral to a physical therapist for what I believed was carpal tunnel syndrome. He listened to my symptoms and said that while he would give me the referral for the splints he also wanted me tested for hypothyroidism. It turned it out I was hypothyroid. The doctor later on said, "I bet you are tired and depressed, and think that's how a new parent should feel." He explained to me about postpartum thyroiditis and Hashimoto's thyroiditis and told me, in my question of when did it start, said he had no way of knowing but he absolutely agreed that my thyroid disease was the cause of my declining milk supply.

Not content to leave it at that, Sharon decided to get the word out about how the onset of low milk supply had coincided with the hypothyroidism:

> I took my best articles to my hospital-based midwife and asked her if she or any of the ob-gyns warn women about thyroid disease in the first year of pregnancy. She admitted they did not and probably should. I commented that the new mother gets lost in the system. If she has had a routine pregnancy and postpartum period, her last visit is six weeks after the baby is born and probably before signs of thyroid disease are noticeable. Monitoring should be done at six-month and one-year periods to see if the new mother is in a hypothyroid or hyperthyroid state. I then contacted the lactation consultant, who proved to be the most open to ideas. When she heard the outcome of my saga, she said, "We always focus on getting the baby to nurse

or to re-establish the mother's milk supply. We never think to have the mother examined."

In my case, my postpartum TSH bounced around like a rubber ball. I went from hyperthyroid immediately postpartum, to the top of the normal range, nearing hypothyroid levels, just weeks later, back to hyperthyroid, and back to hypothyroid, with only tiny dosage adjustments. It appeared that my hormones were fluctuating wildly.

It's well known that the postpartum period can trigger a variety of thyroid and hormonal problems in women who have never had any thyroid problems prior to pregnancy. In someone who is already "hormonally compromised," it's even more likely that the postpartum period can be a period of hormonal upheaval.

Diane was on thyroid hormone replacement for two years before she became pregnant with her third child:

> The obstetrician monitored my thyroid hormones through the pregnancy and the baby was born big and healthy. Shortly after his birth, the symptoms came back in full force. My doctor's office was undergoing staff changes again. I went to one young doctor just out of school. He ran the regular tests and told me they were in the "normal ranges" again. But he did adjust my Synthroid. I was almost down to nothing.

In my case, when Julia was about five months old, I still couldn't shake the major exhaustion, and a gray, depressed feeling that had descended on me about a month after her birth. I went to my regular doctor, sure that I must be suffering from postpartum depression. The doctor, however, decided to run some hormone tests before recommending an antidepressant. It's a good thing she did because she discovered that I had various hormonal imbalances in addition to my thyroid edging out of normal range into hypothyroid TSH levels *again*. She prescribed some natural hormone replacement and changed my thyroid hormone dosage, and soon, it was as if the fog had lifted and the world was a happy place again.

This leads me to another tip I have for hypothyroid mothers. Fairly early on postpartum, pay close attention to symptoms of any hormonal imbalances and have all your hormone levels tested periodically, including thyroid, progesterone, testosterone, and estrogen.

Despite the hormonal ups and downs, I just want to offer hope that you can get pregnant and have a healthy baby while you're being treated for hypothyroidism. I had my wonderful little girl, and she was worth all the hormonal flip-flops in the world! And when it comes to being hypothyroid and having successful pregnancies, you can't get a happier ending than Jeanne's story:

> I have been taking Armour thyroid since I was two years old. I have seven kids, six girls, and one boy. They were all born within ten years. The only problems that I noticed while pregnant was that my thyroid had to be upped to four grains a day. I am now back to taking only one grain a day. My oldest is twenty-three and my youngest is thirteen. Sometimes I wouldn't have minded if my fertility were on the low side!

CHAPTER 12

Hypothyroidism in Infants and Children

*So long as little children are allowed to suffer,
there is no true love in this world.*
ISADORA DUNCAN

Congenital hypothyroidism—hypothyroidism at birth—affects an estimated one in 4,000 newborns. The disease used to be a major cause of mental retardation in children because development of the brain, as well as normal growth of the child, is dependent upon normal levels of thyroid hormone. Now, routine testing for hypothyroidism—usually part of the "heel stick" test given to newborns in the U.S., Canada, and many other nations—has prevented many of the longterm problems that developed due to undetected and untreated hypothyroidism.

It's always worthwhile to verify that your baby has had the newborn-screening tests and that the test screened for congenital hypothyroidism. I remember when I had my baby, I asked the nurses specifically if the heel stick test they were giving her covered hypothyroidism. Not one maternity ward nurse had any idea what the test covered, and I insisted on getting a copy of the state's brochure that explained the test in full. I was relieved to discover that the test did cover hypothyroidism. But, frankly, hospitals aren't perfect, and things can get overlooked; this is one question I recommend everyone ask.

Because congenital hypothyroidism is not that common, it's not always easy to get information about the problem. Typically, when parents or family members contact me regarding a new baby or child's hypothyroidism, I have always referred them to one person:

Kelly Cherkes, who is Thyroid Division Director for the MAGIC Foundation (Major Aspects of Growth In Children) for Children's Growth and Related Adult Disorders. Kelly is an advocate for parents, providing a wealth of information and resources related to infant and childhood hypothyroidism. She is also the mother of a hypothyroid child herself.

According to Kelly, even with the screening program, it's important for parents to watch for the symptoms of congenital hypothyroidism in infants:

    Puffy face, swollen tongue
    Hoarse cry
    Cold extremities, mottled skin
    Low muscle tone (floppy, no strength)
    Poor feeding
    Thick coarse hair that grows low on the forehead
    Large fontanel (soft spot)
    Prolonged jaundice
    Herniated belly button
    Lethargic (lack of energy, sleeps most of the time, appears
        tired even when awake)
    Persistent constipation, bloated, or full to the touch
    Little to no growth

According to Kelly, children with congenital hypothyroidism are usually diagnosed within the first couple weeks of life due to the newborn-screening programs:

> More often than not symptoms are not apparent at birth but can become visible by the time of diagnosis. Most parents feel they have been blessed with a "good" baby because they sleep so much and fuss so little.

When hypothyroidism is discovered in an infant, it is typically due to one of three reasons:

- failure of a normal thyroid gland to function properly;
- a congenital thyroid malformation—including failure to properly develop, position in the wrong location, or undersized; or

- an enzyme defect in iodine metabolism that makes them unable to make thyroid hormone.

Once diagnosis is made, your child should be referred to a pediatric endocrinologist. Kelly has found that for some parents, it can be difficult to find a local pediatric endocrinologist, but even if it means traveling a bit out of your area, it is very important to have your child seen by a specialist at least once. Then, after the pediatric endocrinologist has seen your child, he or she may follow up with your child's pediatrician to ensure proper treatment.

According to Kelly, the doctors should perform other tests to find out more about your child's condition, including a thyroid scan to tell if your child has a thyroid gland or not. Some children have a gland in the wrong place or one that isn't fully developed. This is important because if your child has a gland and it's in the right place the condition may be temporary, what's known as transient hypothyroidism. If your child does not have a gland or the gland is misplaced, your child will need thyroid replacement medication for life. It is good to have this information early on instead of waiting till your child is three, at which point you might have to take her or him off medication unnecessarily to get an accurate scan at that time. Your child will also likely have a bone-age x-ray done. This is an x-ray of the ankle and/or wrist to show the growth of the bones. It is a diagnostic tool used to let doctors know the possible severity of the disorder by determining the time of onset in utero.

In addition to congenital hypothyroidism, children can also develop what's known as "acquired hypothyroidism." Typically, this is hypothyroidism that develops in children due to autoimmune thyroid disease such as Hashimoto's disease. It's more common as children reach puberty or teenage years but still can appear in young children. It is also more common in girls than in boys.

According to Kelly, when children acquire hypothyroidism, it can be more damaging than to an adult. In most instances, when a child develops hypothyroidism it goes unnoticed for quite sometime. Unfortunately, children change so much during childhood that tiredness, mood swings, weight gain, and health problems are often attributed to other causes. Most parents mainly notice the lack of growth. Children who are severely affected due to late diagnosis can lose growth potential along with facing the other health issues that adults also experience.

Kelly believes that people with a family history of hypothyroidism should have their children routinely screened, especially if they test positive for thyroid antibodies. Children who acquire hypothyroidism are treated similarly to those who are born with it. A bone-age and thyroid scan are necessary and very close monitoring of their levels is also a must.

By whatever means your baby or child has become hypothyroid, Kelly recommends that parents keep the results of all tests, along with blood test results and specific values in a journal or record book. Your journal should also include the normal ranges for these tests, so you have a way to gauge where your child falls compared to the normal values. You can use this journal to keep track of the child's symptoms as well, with the goal of becoming familiar with how these levels coincide with your child's health and well-being. Keep in mind that lab levels change depending on your child's age. Once your child reaches twelve, he or she will typically have the same normal ranges as adults.

Treatment for congenital and acquired hypothyroidism involves replacing the missing thyroid hormone in pill form. It is absolutely essential that these pills be taken daily for life because thyroid hormone is critical for all the body's functions. This is *particularly* important for infants and children in order to ensure normal physical, mental, and intellectual development.

When it comes to medication for infants and children, there are various brands of thyroid hormone replacement that can be prescribed. Kelly has some excellent tips that you might want to discuss with your child's doctor:

> For children I recommend the soft pills, Levoxyl or Levothroid. These two dissolve easily in water and crush easily. Synthroid is a very hard pill, which is hard to crush. Then when you add water it clumps up. I found it to be extremely difficult to work with. There is not a liquid form of levothyroxine sodium at present. Some pharmacists will take thirty days of medication, crush the pills, and add them to a "simple syrup," which is administered daily. The problem with this is a po-

tency issue. You don't really know day to day how much hormone your child is receiving because the powder settles and needs vigorous shaking. It's a guess how much each actual dose is. I believe this method, although easier, is not the best for infants.

Kelly has these suggestions for parents on how to give the medication:

1. Dissolve or crush pill in 1 cc of water, breast milk, or milk-based formula. (Do not mix with soy-based formula.) Draw liquid into syringe. Place tip of syringe far back on the inside of infant's cheek and slowly squeeze into child's mouth.

2. Crush pill, wet your finger, roll finger into powder, let baby suck the powdered pill from your finger. This method works the best and ensures the infant gets all the medication.

It is best to administer medication on an empty stomach. It can be difficult with newborns because they feed so frequently. If this is a problem, remember that consistency is the key. It is more important to be consistent in how and when you administer. If there are any kind of malabsorption issues, the blood test will reflect that and your pediatric endocrinologist can adjust the dose accordingly.

When your child is older, around two, he or she can chew the pills instead of having to crush them. Most children like them, and this becomes part of their daily routine.

Normal starting dose for infants is approximately 50 mcg. The goal is to get the child euthyroid (normal thyroid levels) as soon as possible. A child should be clinically and biochemically euthyroid within two to four weeks of treatment. Prolonged hypothyroidism in infancy can cause irreversible brain damage.

According to Kelly, sometimes when older children aren't receiving the proper amount of hormone, they may experience the following symptoms: mood swings, behavioral problems, lack of interests, and poor school performance. It has also been noticed that children with undiagnosed and/or undertreated hypothyroidism are sometimes misdiagnosed with other disorders such as attention deficit hyperactivity disorder (ADD/ADHD). Many children also suffer from upper respiratory infections and have been diagnosed asthmatic until they are on a proper regimen of thyroid replacement hormone.

As your child grows, it is of the utmost importance to keep close track of thyroid levels. Any child who is hypothyroid—congenital or acquired—will need periodic changes in dosage. Doctors often recommend that the child have blood tests at least every six months and even more frequently while an infant. Also, schedule a special thyroid checkup for a girl with hypothyroidism about the time she first begins to menstruate. Hormonal fluctuations may warrant a modification in her thyroid hormone dosage.

With early, proper and regular treatment, your child can grow and develop normally. But keep in mind some additional advice from Kelly:

> Thyroid disorders in children can create a number of symptoms that seem unrelated to the thyroid. As you care for your children, please be aware, it is not just a pill a day. We as parents are the only advocates for our children and empowering ourselves with knowledge of this disorder is the only way we can truly do what's best for them.

CHAPTER 13

Hypothyroidism After Thyroid Cancer

Fall seven times, stand up eight.
JAPANESE PROVERB

In most cases of thyroid cancer, the gland is surgically removed all or in part. For some, the thyroid or any remaining thyroid tissue is ablated using radioactive iodine. The treatment usually results in hypothyroidism, and a lifelong need to be on thyroid hormone replacement.

There are a number of unique issues related to thyroid cancer. These are concerns that are not applicable to people who are hypothyroid due to autoimmune illness or surgical removal or RAI for noncancerous thyroid conditions.

The first unique issue is what is known as TSH suppression, the practice of giving sufficient dosage of thyroid hormone to keep the TSH low, sometimes almost undetectable, in the hyperthyroid range. This is done as a way to prevent thyroid cancer recurrence. Making sure that thyroid cancer survivors are aware of the need for suppression is a mission of Kathy, a thyroid cancer survivor herself. An active member of ThyCa: The Thyroid Cancer Survivors' Association and the associated online email support lists, Kathy has some excellent advice that is very specific to her fellow thyroid cancer survivors:

> If you lost your thyroid gland to thyroid cancer and you believe you have symptoms of hypothyroidism, the most important question is: has your doctor explained to you that in order to prevent recurrence

or spread of papillary or follicular thyroid cancer you must suppress TSH to a below-normal level, meaning that your bloodwork should be more indicative of *hyperthyroidism* than *hypothyroidism*? If your answer is "no," call or fax your doctor as soon as possible.

No doctor ever told me that I was taking Synthroid to do more than replace the functions previously performed by the gland. I had to hear from fellow patients that TSH needed to be suppressed below normal to prevent thyroid cancer recurrence! Ask whether suppression of TSH to a below-normal level has been your doctor's goal, and ask what your TSH is on your current dosage of thyroid replacement hormone. The conservative approach is to suppress TSH below 0.1, but, depending on the circumstances of the case at hand, some endocrinologists will allow TSH of up to 0.3 or 0.5 if the patient feels poorly at lower levels. If, upon talking to your doctor, you learn that your TSH has not been suppressed to below-normal levels, consider either encouraging your doctor to increase your dosage or change to a doctor with more thyroid cancer experience.

The second issue is becoming hypothyroid prior to thyroid scans, or a process sometimes referred to as "going hypo." As part of the process of thyroid cancer followup, periodic scans look for any reappearance of the cancer. Most people are required to stop taking their thyroid hormone and become clinically hypothyroid with elevated TSH levels in the weeks prior to the scan. This is often the most difficult aspect of thyroid cancer follow-up treatment, in that people actually become and remain hypothyroid for weeks in order to ensure the most accurate scan.

Megan, an upbeat young thyroid cancer survivor, has this to say about "going hypo:"

I'm not looking forward to being off the pills because those days will pass slowly, and I'll be feeling pretty bad. Not easy for someone like me who is normally very active and has a to-do list a mile long. Being off the thyroid pills made me absolutely exhausted, like I've been to several all-night parties without the fun. Even my elbows were tired. How do you have tired elbows??? Every day I felt more like a dishrag. I told that to a friend, a psychotherapist, who asked "What color dishrag are you?" I replied "A yellow one, because I am cheerful and positive, even though I feel limp." After that, just thinking about being a yellow dishrag made me smile and feel better. There are days when I can't find the energy to turn on the computer, but when I do, I also sure love to read email jokes. I am keeping my spirits up by laughing. It's good medicine and it doesn't taste bad, except for the tasteless jokes!

Bob, a survivor of papillary thyroid cancer, has some excellent tips gleaned from his two trips to what he calls "Hypoland:"

- Work: Tell your boss ahead of time what to expect and when. When I had a treatment schedule with dates, I followed up with an email.
- Meditate: I realized a month or two ago that I had to get back into meditating. I had learned to meditate when I was in college and over the years since I tried half a dozen or so different techniques. Before I started preparing for the scan, I started meditating twice a day and kept it up while hypo. I really think it helped. Of the techniques I have tried, the best method and the one that has been most widely researched and consistently found effective is Transcendental Meditation. Web site: http://www.tm.org.
- If you start feeling crappy sooner than expected, contact your doctor and see if you can get your TSH level checked early. I was originally scheduled to have blood drawn on the 11th and if my TSH was greater than 40. I would take my tracer dose of RAI on Monday the 14th. As it turned out, I called on Tuesday the 8th and my TSH was 114. I took my 3 mci dose on Wednesday, found I had less than 1 percent uptake on Thursday and a clean scan on Friday the 11th.
- Dealing with other people: When you're hypo, your face will be puffy, your speech will be slurred, and you won't be moving quite as purposefully as normal. As a result, it is likely strangers will respond to you differently than you're used to. I found myself "under observation" at the library and in a couple of stores. I'm also afraid I scared a lady at my daughter's pre-school.

When thyroid cancer survivors "go hypo," doctors typically target a fairly elevated TSH level for the scan. Getting to a TSH of

30 or 40, or over 100 as Bob described, can mean more than your fair share of fullscale hypothyroid symptoms. It makes sense not to plan important, stressful, or taxing events during this period, and to avoid taking on too much during this time.

With both practicality and wit, Bob also offers the following list of the top ten things you should *never* do while hypo, compiled from his and other experiences, "not all of which are mine," as he says:

Ten Things You Should NEVER Do While Hypo

10. Ask for a raise

9. Go on a first date

8. Go on a second date

7. Install gas appliances

6. Give your daughter a haircut

5. Use your real name when calling a radio talk show

4. Learn to jet ski

3. Start remodeling your kitchen

2. Meet your future in-laws

1. Apply for a hand gun purchase permit

Ric Blake is a thyroid cancer survivor and the dedicated founder and organizer of the first Thyroid Cancers Survivors Conference, which was known as ThyCa '98, and one of the founders of the Thyroid Cancer Survivors' Association. Ric has some light-hearted—but quite valid—ideas to share as well, in his "Tips for Thyroid Cancer Survivors While Hypothyroid:"

In hypo-hell, one is much like a cat, an old and cranky cat. For those preparing to go off your hormones in preparation for a body scan, we offer this guide for you and your significant other.

- As with any old cat, hugs and snuggles works wonders.
- As with any cranky cat, keeping your distance is a smart idea.
- Change the balance of household responsibilities: Your partner can take on more; you can sleep.
- Add more physical activity to your schedule: Your partner can rub your back; you can purr.

- Consider separate vacations: Your partner can go to Hawaii; you can go someplace warm.
- Divide up household chores: Your partner can do them all; you can sleep.
- Reschedule cooking responsibilities: Your partner can go out; you can eat salt-free between naps.
- Change your recreation schedule: Your partner can go dancing; you can keep the bed warm.
- Rent videos. Your partner can rent *Fatal Attraction 2*; you can rent *Sleeping Beauty*.
- Rethink making major decisions: Make no decision more complicated than which shoe to put on first.

Ric has also developed what he refers to as "the more serious version:"

Forewarned is forearmed has much merit for thyca survivors. In the three and a half years since my diagnosis and surgery, I've had body scans and RAI four times. On average, I've been hypothyroid every ten months, making me a reluctant expert on journeys to hypo-hell and back. The last two times have been easier because by 1997 I had met other survivors and learning from others' experiences is the best resource we have for living well with thyca.

My doctors told me I would feel increasingly worse as I became more and more hypothyroid. What they didn't tell me was just *how* much worse I would feel. If they had, I would have been better able to plan my life. Each time I followed the same sequence: six weeks off hormones, scan, RAI, then begin hormones four days or so after the radiation. Here are the survival tips I've learned along the way.

- Working: If possible, don't work full time the last week before and the first week after your scan. Use your vacation time and plan lots of naps. If you must work, negotiate with your employer and work half-days if possible.
- During this two-week period, don't:
  - drive a car
  - operate dangerous equipment
  - sign important papers
  - make significant decisions

start a new job

move to a new house or apartment

tell your boss what you really think

- Avoid:

stressful conversations

difficult people

malls

rush-hour commuting, even if you're sitting on the passenger's side of the car

- Put off:

working on important projects

anything requiring clear thinking and organizational skill

everything that can be put off

- Do:

drink lots of water to prevent constipation

eat lots of fruits and vegetables for the same reason

exercise even when you don't feel like it

cut down on calories to avoid weight gain

plan on being very good to yourself; buy yourself something special

plan on seeing lots of movies, plays, and concerts that require *no* thinking on your part

buy new batteries for the television remote: channel surfing is therapeutic

weed your garden *before* you're severely hypo

- Expect to:

be very cold; carry a sweater at all times, even in the summer

be a jerk to the people around you; apologize ahead of time

lose your car and house keys often

forget the names of your spouse and children

get lost driving familiar roads

- When preparing for scans, you should:

wear warm clothes (sweats are best) and take a blanket

if possible, take a portable radio, tape, or CD player

Not everyone has a fullscale reaction to the hypothyroid period before a scan. Margie found that despite being off her thyroid hormone for a total of more than five weeks and reaching a TSH of 95, she didn't suffer hypothyroidism symptoms throughout the entire period. Her symptoms only began a few days before she was due to start back on her thyroid hormone replacement. She has some theories about why she didn't experience the full brunt of "going hypo:"

> I attribute this to serious workouts, mainly weights and stationary gym bike, at least five days a week, which I started over four months ago. I was doing five miles a day on the bike. The symptoms I have experienced are quick sudden weight gain—15 pounds in two weeks—problems concentrating and being irritated at things that do not normally bother me much. Also sudden exhaustion, then rebounding.

It's important to mention Thyrogen to thyroid cancer survivors, a product approved in 1998. Thyrogen allows some patients to avoid the process of withdrawal from thyroid hormone replacement. Patients switch from their thyroid hormone replacement to Thyrogen prior to the scan, and don't suffer the experience of going hypothyroid. It's certainly something to discuss with your doctor. Thyrogen is a very expensive drug and only certain patients are good candidates. It is not as reliable as the full hormone withdrawal/ "going hypo" process, but it is considered useful for those patients who have had several clear scans, and thus limited likelihood of cancer recurrence.

A third issue is the low-iodine diet. Many patients are required to go on a low-iodine diet for at least two weeks before the scan to ensure the greatest accuracy. This diet increases the reliability of the test. Doctors often ask patients to continue the diet through the testing procedure and during any subsequent treatment with radioactive iodine, so some people can be on it for a number of weeks.

While you should get specifics from your doctor regarding the low-iodine diet, it's basically fine to eat fresh meats, fresh poultry, fresh or frozen vegetables, fresh fruits, as long as you don't cook with or add specific condiments and other foodstuffs that contain iodine. So, generally, here are the low-iodine diet guidelines:

- *Avoid iodized salt and salty foods:* You'll want to avoid all iodized salt and sea salt products as well. You can use non-iodized salt, Kosher salt is non-iodized, for example. Be aware that most salty foods like pretzels, chips, popcorn, and nuts may have iodized salt, so you should avoid them. Also, most restaurant and fast foods contain salt, and there's no way to determine which outside salt is iodized. Your best bet is to avoid most salty foods and restaurants.

- *Avoid seafood:* Fish, shellfish, seaweed, and kelp are all high in iodine.

- *Avoid dairy products:* Including milk, ice cream, cheese, cream, yogurt, butter, egg yolks, and milk chocolate. The only exception is egg whites and chocolate made without milk.

- *Avoid foods with the following additives:* Carrageen, agar, algin, alginates.

- *Avoid cured, corned, or spicy meats:* Avoid bacon, ham, sausage, salami, lox, corned beef, sauerkraut, etc. Fresh meat is acceptable.

- *Avoid commercial bakery products:* Since commercial baked goods often contain iodine, you'll need to have only homemade or local bakery products.

- *Avoid vitamins and food supplements:* If they contain iodine—and most multivitamins do—you'll need to stop taking them.

- *Avoid red, orange or brown food, pills, and capsules:* Many red, red-orange, and brown food dyes contain iodine.

- *Avoid other foods that may contain iodine dyes and preservatives:* These include soy products—like soy sauce, tofu, and soy milk—molasses, instant coffee and tea, canned fruits and vegetables.

While we don't have the space to present menu ideas and all the various tips and tricks used by thyroid cancer patients to make food interesting on the low-iodine diet, we do have a few excellent tips from Bob to help you follow the guidelines.

Start shopping for staples ahead of time. I had a little trouble finding margarine with neither salt nor dairy this year. The supermarket that carried Fleishman's version last year now carries Mother's. Some stores I tried don't carry any. All the supermarkets I checked had non-iodized salt next to the regular salt. I found salt-free peanut butter in the dietetic food section.

Try a few days on the diet before you're hypo. That way, you'll find out what does and doesn't work while you still have your wits about you and can do something about it. You also won't find yourself, as I did last year, standing in the middle of Best Buy, hypo and hungry with heavy metal blaring while you're trying to pick out a bread machine.

Get a vegan cookbook. Vegans don't use any eggs or dairy. They also don't use much salt, so don't be surprised if things taste pretty bland at first. You can always add non-iodized "salt and pepper to taste" after you cooked it. I was amazed at the difference between my first and second bite of vegan chili. Another good source is the Vegetarian Resource Group (Web site: http://www.vrg.org). Their recipes aren't all vegan, but they do give directions for things like mixing cashews and water in a blender to substitute for milk in cooking. (i.e., "1 cup raw cashews, 3 cups water, blend both for 5 minutes and refrigerate. Shake well before use.")

Don't view this as an opportunity to lose weight, go vegetarian, or make any other dietary changes not related to iodine. You're going through enough. Do try to notice if you're allergic to dairy. I seem to be. My nose stopped running about a week into the diet and started again shortly after eating pizza last night."

A fourth issue is related to thyroid hormone replacement. While the T4 versus T3 drug battle wages on between conventional and complementary practitioners and their patients, nowhere is the battle fiercer than when it comes to the issue of thyroid cancer suppression.

Most doctors treating thyroid cancer survivors are adamant in their insistence that levothyroxine is the only drug of choice for thyroid cancer suppression and feel that there is absolutely no role for the T4/T3 synthetic or natural drugs as part of management of thyroid cancer. They have a concern that there may be ups and downs in TSH levels due to the use of T3, and that even small fluctuations in TSH could fail to prevent cancer recurrence.

I'll be honest here. I don't know if there's definitive proof that taking added T3 or a drug with T3 is or isn't a problem with thyroid suppression or increases the risk of recurrence. I haven't seen research reports that definitely say "yes" or "no." Ultimately, what thyroid hormone replacement you take for thyroid cancer suppression and how you feel on that drug is an extremely important matter for you to take up with your doctor. Just keep in mind that in terms of the right treatment and program for total wellness, each patient is ultimately an individual, and some doctors recognize this more than others.

Gail is a sixty-year-old woman, who has lived half her life as a thyroid cancer survivor and now provides support to newly diagnosed thyroid cancer patients. Bucking the convention, she takes Armour thyroid, prescribed by her conventional doctor. Gail found that, unlike today, there was little information available to her when she was diagnosed in 1968. Now she is active in the medical community and well informed about thyroid disease. Even more so since becoming active on the Internet.

> I never knew there were issues with T3 replacement. I had no idea that the endocrinology community frowned on the use of Armour thyroid or, for that matter, any replacement with a T3/T4 combination. Although I had a very active and potentially fatal situation in my battle with thyroid cancer, I have been on a T3/T4 drug for 27 of the last 31 years.
>
> I recently asked my endocrinologist how can it be that I survived, against some steep odds, on a drug that was supposed to be inadequate for suppression and not good for me? His reply, though not

completely to the point, indicated his flexibility against the T4-only theory. And then he said, "You feel good don't you? We are not going to fool with success!" On the whole my endocrinologist does not advocate the use of T3. But in my situation he stands firm. I hardly ever experienced the dilemmas that patients go through with their T4 medication. My TSH suppression came right in on target through all the years. The "bounce" that we hear about with T3 never was apparent in my blood testing. The variable times and circumstances when that blood was taken over the years are many. It makes me wonder why T3 is not looked at a bit differently by the medical community.

The final issue is general wellness after thyroid cancer. At low TSH levels, thyroid cancer survivors can experience symptoms of hyperthyroidism, and even though TSH is suppressed, at times, hypothyroidism. While some symptoms are no doubt due to the thyroid, there can also be a tendency to attribute most health problems to the underlying thyroid issues.

Again, Kathy feels that if your TSH is being adequately suppressed, but you are still having symptoms, you'll need to look at some other issues.

Have you talked to your primary care doctor or a counselor as well as your endocrinologist about your symptoms? Perhaps there is a valid medical reason for your symptoms that is totally unrelated to your thyroid cancer and hormone suppression therapy. Perhaps there is other bloodwork that should be ordered. Perhaps the fears and uncertainty related to a cancer diagnosis have led to anger, depression, or other emotional trauma for which psychotherapy is indicated.

Kathy also feels that it may be important to have a partnership with an endocrinologist in which you feel comfortable suggesting alternative or unconventional approaches to thyroid hormone suppression therapy.

If you have ruled out any causes other than thyroid suppression therapy for your hypothyroid-like symptoms, then explore the feasibility of working with your endocrinologist to modify the current approach to alleviate the symptoms. Perhaps, if you have had a history of negative scans and favorable Tg readings, your doctor would be willing to lower your thyroid hormone dosage slightly and allow your TSH to rise. Perhaps, if you are taking only levothyroxine, your doctor would be willing to add supplemental T3 or switch to a T4/T3 combination.

Kathy also feels that one of the more frustrating aspects of thyroid cancer aftercare is the fact that, if your care is properly managed, you will never again have a "normal" level of thyroid hormone in your system.

Remember, you are different than someone with thyroid disease. While the thyroid disease patient strives to attain normal thyroid hormone levels, you are striving for optimal adaptation to abnormal levels. The payoff is increased odds of avoiding recurrence or spread of your thyroid cancer.

Suppressed TSH levels mean that you may have to pay more attention, or take a different approach to things like diet, exercise, relaxation, or supplements than you did before having your thyroid removed. Kathy suggests taking advantage of all the information available at the library, bookstore, on the Internet, or in patient/survivor support groups to develop a customized, individual program for adapting to the reality of TSH suppression. Just be sure to keep in touch with your doctor about the approach you develop, and get bloodwork done soon enough after any major dietary changes to ensure that your TSH remains adequately suppressed.

Long-term thyroid cancer survivor Gail has some thoughts about life with and after thyroid cancer:

My journey with thyroid cancer was tumultuous in the early years when I had five major surgeries in four years. Since then I have lived an active, healthy life, raising three wonderful children and doing volunteer work with cancer patients. Cancer became a stepping stone to a better life and understanding of what is important. I put the fears behind me and let the joys of life become my focal point.

PART IV

LIVING WELL NOW
AND IN THE FUTURE

CHAPTER 14

Living Well with Hypothyroidism

Drugs are not always necessary, but belief in recovery always is.
NORMAN COUSINS

For most of us, there's no single magic pill that ensures that we can live well with hypothyroidism. Rather, the secret is an approach that blends the science *and* the art of living well.

Hopefully, this book has already provided enough information to help you get on the right thyroid hormone replacement at the right dosage for you. This is essential to living well. The *science* of living well also relies on resolving any other hormonal or chemical imbalances and health issues that might get in the way of being well and living well. For this, a productive partnership with caring, smart healthcare practitioners will take you a long way.

The *art* of living well opens up a whole additional world of opportunities. You can find the right alternative therapies and integrate them into your overall treatment, learn to develop a positive attitude, choose foods to nourish mind and body, or learn how to empower yourself to move forward on your own behalf.

Ultimately, your success begins with a fundamental belief in your own recovery. Yes, hypothyroidism may not be the easiest condition to completely resolve, and, yes, many doctors may not invest much energy in the problem . . . but leave that behind. *You* must have faith and believe that *you* can recover and go on to live well.

This chapter looks at some various approaches to help you live well. These ideas mainly come from the best possible source: people living well with hypothyroidism themselves. Some advice comes from doctors and healthcare practitioners who have demonstrated their ability to help people live well. You'll find many ideas to consider as part of your own effort to live well.

An endocrinologist, T'ai Chi, and a vegetarian diet might be the answer for one person. Or the addition of a T3 drug, aerobic exercise, and participation in a chronic disease support group at the local hospital may work for another. Each person's optimal approach is likely to be different. Your job is to find the mix of ideas that works best for *you*.

In my case, for example, I've found that a holistic doctor, the addition of T3, periodic acupuncture, yoga, light exercise like walking, a low-glycemic diet, online support, a nutritionist advising me on vitamins, supplements and diet, and a sense of humor constitute the best mix for me.

Sherry Ann has found an approach that works for her:

> I pray a lot and I thank the Lord that I am where I am today and that I am not as I was years ago. I really thought then that I was going to die. I believe humor is great. It keeps our spirits up, and we need to laugh because Lord knows I have shed my share of tears. Learn all you can about this, and if your doctor doesn't understand, you find another one. Keep prayer in your life. Try to find a support group to go to and take your family with you.

It's also useful to identify a philosophy, so to speak, about dealing with your hypothyroidism. For some people, this philosophy is actually expressed in the form of a metaphor. Megan, a thyroid cancer survivor who also loves whitewater rafting, adopted her good friend's advice:

> She told me that she views my health like river rafting. When there is whitewater, try to stay in the boat, avoid the suckholes, and know there is always a way to eddy out after a while. Meantime, you keep moving down the river and around the bends. It helps when you have a good crew in your boat . . . like friends.

Ted also has a metaphor to describe his philosophy of hypothyroidism:

> Driving on snow or ice is no problem whatsoever. Piece of cake. That is, until you need to change lanes, change speed, make a turn, or have to swerve to avoid hitting a pig in the road. It's not the everyday occurrences that affect our thyroid balance, it is trying to change something else that gets us in trouble.

As you read through the various suggestions on living well with hypothyroidism, I hope you find ideas about approaches that might work for you. And as you read the ideas and hopes of other thyroid patients, give some thought to what you'd like *your* personal philosophy to be.

My personal philosophy is that even if I can't resolve every single thing about my hypothyroidism, I keep looking for the answers I can find. This makes me feel I have some control over the situation. Along the way, I even try to have a laugh or two! And I find great comfort in sharing whatever information I have with others.

LIVING WELL TIP #1:
FIND THE RIGHT HYPOTHYROIDISM THERAPY

There's no doubt that the right therapy for hypothyroidism is a basic requirement for living well. No amount of Synthroid is going to solve your problem, if what you really will thrive on is Armour. You can add time-released T3 therapy to your Levoxyl, but that won't help if you don't need the added T3 and start to feel jittery. Finding the right drug at the right dosage is not an automatic process for everyone, and may require a bit of experimenting and patience while your doctor finetunes and tweaks your thyroid hormone regimen.

When I was first diagnosed, my doctor put me on Thyrolar. A year later, after reading all the medical literature and initially buying into the marketing spiels, I told the doctor I wanted to go on Synthroid. She reluctantly agreed. Within a month, my hair started falling out rapidly, and a thyroid test showed that I'd become hyper-thyroid on an equivalent dose. My dose was reduced slightly, the hair loss increased, and I developed an ovarian cyst. Another TSH test a month later showed that I had become hypothyroid. Back to hyperthyroid, then hypothyroid again. After four more months of wildly fluctuating TSH levels, and further hair loss, we decided to go back to Thyrolar. Things calmed down right away. My doctor and I didn't need any medical textbook or double-blind study to tell us that I did better on Thyrolar than Synthroid. You may have to go though this process periodically, but it's worth it to ensure you're getting the right medicine and dosage you need.

LIVING WELL TIP #2:
FIND A GREAT DOCTOR (AND
GET RID OF A BAD ONE)

The right doctor is an important—almost essential—part of living well. You probably can live well *despite* your doctor, if you truly have no option but to work with an HMO doctor you're stuck with, or the only endocrinologist within 500 miles. When you have a choice, however, one of the most important things you can do is find a great doctor and leave the bad ones behind.

Renee is one patient who needed to find a more positive doctor to help her live well:

> I like to be an informed medical consumer. My doctor claimed to be okay with it. Then, I started having some chest pains. I have read that when taking thyroid hormones, chest pains can be a serious concern. When I saw my doctor to get a refill on my thyroid prescription, I told him that I've been having some chest pains. He listened to my heart and called me a "neurotic fruitcake." No kidding . . . his exact words! He said it several times. I refused to respond. I just wanted to get out of that office! I am looking for a new doctor. I am not a "fruitcake" and I highly doubt that I am "neurotic." I think a doctor needs to listen to (even unfounded) concerns and reassure patients (even "neurotic" ones) without humiliation. I have lost trust and he has lost a patient!"

In her path toward wellness, Geri also found it was time for a new doctor:

The primary care physician (PCP) who diagnosed me has since been fired (by me) because she had a *horrible* attitude. She never answered my questions, didn't take my concerns seriously, generally acted like she had no time for me, and treated me like an uninformed idiot, which I'm definitely not. I'm a health/medical/science writer on a TV science news show, so I deal with this type of information every day. I found another PCP on a referral from friends, and so far so good.

Bill is quite an expert on doctors, after being disabled for many years as a result of military activity:

I've learned to classify doctors as one, excellent, two, satisfactory, and three, *get lost!* During the past fifty-some years, I have watched the infiltration of the "Hallowed Halls of Hippocrates" by the incompetent, the mercenaries, and the prestige- and ego-seekers. I have also discovered that a successful doctor/patient relationship is as dependent on me, the patient, as it is on the doctor. It is up to me to search until I find a competent doctor who can earn my confidence.

Sometimes, you'll find a fresh perspective after changing doctors. For years, Yobeth's regular physician conducted an annual blood test for her hypothyroidism and never changed her dose. Yobeth decided to start seeing an endocrinologist:

As it turned out, my medication needed adjusting. However, while I was there I learned a lot that I'd never known. I learned there were links to thyroid disease, diabetes, and high cholesterol. This came as a total shock. I'd never been told [that] or checked [for it] by any of my other doctors. I do have high cholesterol and my three-month average glucose test was high, but I'm not diabetic yet. Maybe I'm overreacting, but it seems doctors should take this a little more seriously and also educate patients more thoroughly.

Personally, I have to say that I am extremely lucky, in that I have a wonderful doctor who is my partner in the search for wellness. My physician, Kate Lemmerman, M.D., has these thoughts about the key characteristics of her patients who live well with a chronic and, sometimes, debilitating and exhausting condition like hypothyroidism:

> The key characteristic to living well with any chronic condition is setting the stage for healing in your life. You try to provide ideal conditions for the body to heal. And what we need for those ideal conditions is a combination of proper nutrition, appropriate exercise, and a healthy mental attitude. I think it is very helpful to find a physician whom you trust and with whom you can communicate. Even if they are not "experts" in the field, if they are dedicated to your well-being, they will learn along with you the best way to enhance your health.

Dr. Lemmerman's point is valid. She is not an endocrinologist or thyroid expert. But she is always learning, always trying to keep up with new information and is a talented, open-minded, and caring physician, who practices medicine as an art. She is dedicated to my well-being, and you can't ask for anything more.

Chapter 6 offered a number of tips on how to find a doctor and communicate well with him or her. If you have doubts about your current doctor, don't forget that your doctor works for you, and just like a plumber or accountant, if your doctor isn't doing a good job or treats you like a second-class citizen, it's time to shop around.

LIVING WELL TIP #3:
EDUCATE YOURSELF ABOUT
HYPOTHYROIDISM AND HEALTH

I can't emphasize enough how important it is for you to really understand hypothyroidism. So often, people contact me, complaining that they don't feel well after a year or more on Synthroid, and ask "What should I do?" When I ask them what their TSH level is, they say "What level? I don't know about this. I just want to feel well." Inevitably, it turns out that they are high-normal, or even clinically hypothyroid, or have an extremely low T3 level, and a discussion with the doctor allows for some dosage modifications or a change in medication, and they are feeling better soon.

If you don't feel well, you simply can't afford to say "I don't know—or want to know—about this." You *must* take it upon yourself to understand what's going on, so you can ask the right questions, discuss options with your doctor, and find another doctor if yours doesn't make sense.

Allyson has this to say about the need for self-education:

> Doctors who see five patients an hour do not have time for explanations and questions. Thyroid patients must learn and ask questions, due to the very nature of this illness. I obtained the information I possess today from two sources: books written by patients and doctors, as well as the Internet.

Megan, a thyroid cancer survivor, prides herself on being knowledgeable about her health issues:

> Read everything you can get your hands on. Knowledge is power. The more informed you are, the less fear you have. Do whatever you can to feel you have some power in an out-of-control situation. Even if that only means learning more about your disease or its treatments. Know that you have choices.

Geri, a health-and-science writer and TV producer, has this to say about dealing with doctors:

> Most of my conflicts with doctors have arisen because I'm a very good researcher and have medical/science background that lets me investigate things more than most patients do. Most docs don't like it when you demonstrate that you have actual knowledge about something. And, frankly, I think this is the fault of patients almost as much as it is of the doctors . . . most patients blindly accept what a physician tells them and consider themselves too dumb to know otherwise. So when informed patients like us come along, the docs have no idea what to do with us!

Toy Lin felt that lack of information could have meant better health for her over the years:

> Had I had a doctor who explained all of this to me years ago, I would not have gone through all of this. I was never told what symptoms to look for. Thanks to my husband, who is very supportive, I got a computer. Otherwise I would still be in the dark about this disease. I was totally amazed at the information available, information the doctors neglected to give me. I realize now I have to take control of my life and not put all of my trust in the doctors.

Who knows what developments may be announced tomorrow regarding hypothyroidism? And who knows when—or even if—your doctor will hear about those developments? The Resources chapter in the Appendix of this book includes many useful Web sites, newsletters, books, and practitioners to help you educate yourself. If you want to live well, your responsibility is to be aware of available options. You can't afford not to stay up-to-date because you just might miss hearing about a new drug or new therapy that could be the answer for you.

LIVING WELL TIP #4:
HELP EDUCATE OTHERS

One important thing everyone with hypothyroidism can do is help educate others and correct common misconceptions about the condition.

Few people know much about hypothyroidism, beyond unfairly characterizing it as "a disease that makes middle-aged women fat." This unfair, inaccurate characterization is part of the reason the disease is so often overlooked and underdiagnosed by doctors, and why there is so little interest in finding better treatments and cures. Part of living well is making sure that others understand and doing your part to raise awareness.

Sometimes, education starts at home. Probably the most appalling letter I've ever received was from the husband of a woman newly diagnosed with hypothyroidism. This unsupportive man was clearly in the dark about the condition:

> Is there really such a thing as a thyroid disease? Is it contagious? The women on my wife's side of the family all seem to have it. Is it hereditary? Does my wife's lack of ambition and motivation have anything to do with it . . . or is it simply the result of this "so called" disease? Will she be more ambitious or self-motivated if she takes Synthroid?

Honestly, I felt for his wife. Hypothyroidism seemed the least of her problems. But after sending him extensive information about hypothyroidism, he actually wrote back to say that he was trying to be more patient and understanding with his wife. So perhaps even *he* was capable of being "educated!"

Cathy's story shows how critical it is to help educate others about hypothyroidism:

> When I learned that I had hypothyroidism I told my mother. Her reaction was "Oh, I know something about that from my friend Sally. It made her lazy." This, of course, angered me—that my mother would imply that people with hypothyroidism are lazy. There's a big difference in being a lazy person and being tired because you have a disease.

When you encounter lack of understanding or misconceptions, take the time to explain the situation. One woman said that she was so convinced that some of her co-workers were suffering from hypothyroidism that she filled them in on the symptoms and convinced nine of them to be tested. Amazingly, six of the nine were hypothyroid, with TSH levels ranging from 18 to the hundreds. A little education can go a long way toward helping others.

LIVING WELL TIP #5:
BE BOTH PATIENT *AND* PERSISTENT

"Patient" is a confusing word. The word patient derives from a Latin verb, which means "to suffer." According to the dictionary, patient, as an adjective, means putting up with pain or provocation without complaint. The noun refers to an individual awaiting or under medical care and treatment, or "one that is acted upon." I'm not going to suggest that you should be a "patient patient," putting up with pain without complaint while you are "acted upon" by doctors! Rather, I prefer another definition: "remaining steadfast despite opposition, difficulty, or adversity."

You may need patience just to get through the diagnosis process, much less the search for effective treatment. During the years she tried to get diagnosed, Cathi kept a journal, which helped her hang on to hope:

> Each day I would write out "SURVIVAL" on the top of the page and list the things I'd have to do to make it through the day with the pain, the fatigue, holding-on-to-furniture just to stand up. I would list the things I was going to do when my mystery problem was cured and simply fantasize about a future free of pain and what that would be like.

With diagnosis and treatment of her hypothyroidism, Cathi was able to stop fantasizing, move beyond just surviving, and start really living well.

Even with the best therapies or the right drug, you can't expect miracles overnight, so patience is essential at all stages of treatment. But patience doesn't mean inaction. One of the hardest aspects of a chronic condition like hypothyroidism is the need to be both patient *and* persistent at the same time. You can't give up trying to find the right answers, the right doctor, or the right treatment.

Toy Lin is someone who has decided to persist in her search for answers regarding her health:

> I am still struggling with fatigue, migraines, dry skin, muscle pain, concentration problems, memory loss, thin fingernails, and allergies. I am hopeful these things will improve. I am working with my family doctor to get my levels down to where I feel well. If he won't continue on that path, then I will keep looking for a doctor who will treat me by the symptoms and not the lab numbers. I'm tired of sitting on the

sidelines and watching the parade go by. I want quality of life. I won't give up until I get it back.

Carol, a fifty-two-year-old woman with hypothyroidism, feels that patience and perseverance are the words that best depict her experience with hypothyroidism.

> Patience to wait for the slow response of the medication. Perseverance to go back for repeated blood tests. Patience with myself when I can't do anything after working all day. Perseverance to search for a new GP doctor after finding out from that my GP didn't know how to read the lab results and had not treated my hypothyroidism. Patience to wait for two-and-a-half months to get in to see a top endocrinologist. Perseverance to make up all the time I missed at work to go to doctors and labs. Patience with insensitive friends and co-workers. Perseverance with doctors that prescribed tests that were detrimental or inappropriate after telling them I was hypothyroid.

Susan perfectly sums it up when she says: "It is so frustrating that when you are feeling your worst you have to fight the hardest." But that is exactly the point. Living with a chronic disease is a marathon, not a 100-yard dash. Hypothyroidism is one of those "slow and steady wins the race" situations.

LIVING WELL TIP #6:
SURROUND YOURSELF WITH PERSONAL SUPPORT

One aspect of living well with any chronic disease is surrounding yourself with supportive people. Spouses, family members, friends, children, coworkers, support group members—all can play a part in helping to encourage your return to good health. The last thing you need is someone who doesn't believe you are ill, makes fun of you, or doesn't cut you some slack when you're not feeling well.

Rachel, a woman in her early twenties, emphasizes the importance of the right kind of friends and support in her life:

I have discovered who my true friends are, as some believe I'm "being ill" just to get attention. I've actually realized my priorities are to take care of myself—and to get much more sleep than I used to! Needless to say, I've lost several friends, just because I couldn't go out at night with them. While that hurts, I realize there are better friends out there, friends who support me. My boyfriend and I had only started dating when I first got sick, so I said to him, "I don't know how long I'll be sick for, but you may leave now," and he told me I was being silly. He has stuck by me. . . .

Some of the best spouses and friends are those who take the time to understand hypothyroidism, so they can understand you. Tom has this recommendation for spouses and partners of people with hypothyroidism:

Go to the doctor, ask questions, and find out what they are going through. It will make those times when they seem unbearable understandable, and understanding and love from you is the best medicine they can get . . . and the quickest.

It's very important to open up and share your experiences with others. Renee had this to say about the importance of personal support:

I hope that fellow patients have and rely on a strong personal support network. The reason I say this is that when I was hypo and depressed . . . I didn't even have the self-esteem to tell my husband how bad it was for me. The isolation was part of the depression for me. . . . not a good thing at all. I got myself into a place where I felt very alone. It was weird, and it took several weeks to get back to feeling like myself again after I started my thyroxine.

If, like Renee, you don't feel comfortable talking to your spouse or partner, it's worthwhile discussing your situation with someone else. If you're not comfortable talking with family and friends, consider seeing a therapist for a few visits, or get online where you can remain anonymous while you exchange information, support, and camaraderie with others going through similar experiences.

Personally, my husband has always been interested in understanding more about hypothyroidism, and has been extremely supportive. I also found tremendous support by participating at alt.support.thyroid, the online newsgroup. I was amazed to find other people dealing with the same thyroid concerns I had and really enjoyed the interchange, benefiting from information and support.

Ted, a fellow alt.support.thyroid friend, also feels strongly about his participation in the online alt.support.thyroid group:

> It is an outlet to help others get support and has been an inlet to get feedback for my own use. There is a lot more information out there than any *one* person can assimilate. That includes doctors. If thyroid conditions represent about 5 percent of the population, it just isn't likely that any *one* doctor has seen all the complications that often occur.

In recent years, while keeping in touch with people like Ted, I've turned to the community at my own thyroid bulletin board. This is an active group of people with thyroid problems who provide mutual support and information, spiced up with a sense of humor and a great deal of compassion. I never fail to find a smile, or an uplifting story, or some empathetic grumbling when I need it.

The value of support is never so great as when we discover that friends know us better than we do at times. Joyce found this out when her hypothyroidism took a turn for the worse.

> When I hit menopause, my thyroid became the roller-coaster ride from hell. Up, down, and all around, sometimes with dramatic drops within a two-week span. Not understanding why, my family physician would increase and decrease my medications, hoping to get me level. After a gentle push, or perhaps a shove in this case, by a dear friend, Rosy, I finally decided I needed to take control of my own body. Rosy didn't beat around the bush when she said, "I am very concerned for you. I want my friend Joyce back, you need to pursue other options and take control of your body and your life, whatever it takes!" Rosy had her sharpshooter aimed, but she backed off when I promised her I would begin researching my disease, looking for clues. In despera-

tion, I began doing research on the Web, all the while giving Rosy intermittent reports on my progress. In my research, I read somewhere on the Web that some vitamins or other prescription medications might interfere with the absorption of thyroid replacement medications. With this ammunition, I asked my family practice physician for a consult to an endocrinologist to solve this mystery.

After a thorough examination and a few questions, the endocrinologist, with a few simple directions, turned my upside-down life around. "Take your vitamins and other prescription medications in the morning and your Synthroid at night." In my case, when I stopped taking my hormone medication for six days each month, my level would shoot back up again, thereby explaining why I consistently went up and down.

My recovery was very dramatic. Within days, I began remembering things; I felt like working out again, I was smiling, happy, and creative. In other words, Joyce was back! I am happy to report that several months later, Rosy's friend, Joyce, is as feisty and tenacious as she once was, full of vim, vigor, and a little vinegar on the side. Thank you, my friend.

The message here? Every person with hypothyroidism needs a Rosy—a supportive friend, spouse, family member, or even cyberpal. Treasure each and every Rosy in your life!

LIVING WELL TIP #7:
DON'T BE AFRAID TO STICK UP FOR YOURSELF

The buzzword for this is "empowerment," but let's call it what it is—being able to stick up for yourself with doctors and medical professionals. This is an absolutely essential skill for anyone with a chronic health problem because you're going to spend some time with health practitioners. No point wasting time and money being lectured at or cowed by your doctor. Learn to stick up for yourself, speak up, and say your peace.

Carla, a woman in her early fifties with hypothyroidism, has some thoughts about being an empowered patient:

When I had to start on replacement therapy, I was, of course, given Synthroid. I felt terrible on this medication and my blood pressure, normally quite low, shot through the roof. My doctor was baffled. While researching, I found that a certain number of the general public has a metabolism that does not convert synthetic T4 to T3 when the brain calls for it. I asked my doctor to prescribe Cytomel. He did, and I felt much, much better. If I had not had the capability and resources to investigate this matter on my own, I shudder to think where I would be today. I feel that no matter what doctor you are seeing or what his credentials are, you are sunk if you do not take a very active role in your own healthcare in general and thyroid treatment in particular.

Tom has some unique advice from the man's perspective:

The most important thing to remember, man or woman, is that you alone are in charge of your body, and you must not ever let anyone, no matter how many degrees, *not* keep you informed and involved. Take one day at a time, allow your spouse to help, and ask for help, too. Both are problems men seem to have. This disorder and our modern-day beliefs about "what makes a man" conflict with each other in the worst sort of way. Your life is not worth being macho over.

Peg, a teacher, has realized that it isn't always simple to be an empowered patient. She's tapping her desire to be well as a motivator:

I have a master's degree and am currently undergoing postgraduate training that I will apply to my doctorate, which I plan to pursue and obtain. Yet nobody has listened to me. Blame it on doctors not taking women seriously or what have you. The bottom line is: I neglected some of my own power by allowing myself to be "talked out" of my feelings, intuition, and instincts. But I'm taking that power back, empowering *myself* and advocating for myself by collecting information to support me. Yes, I am passionate about this. This is my *life*, and I believe (hope and pray) that it won't be too long until I get it *back*!! No more passive role for this lady. I'm climbing over from the back seat I've been in and taking over the driving. And I *will not stop* until I find the doctor who has the expertise to help me. I'm not cured yet, but I haven't felt this good in *years*. Hope is a very powerful motivator. Everyone deserves to have his or her health.

Toy Lin has her own excellent ten-point program for dealing with hypothyroidism that illustrates how an empowered patient can take charge of her own healthcare:

1. Educate yourself, read, and print out as much as possible.
2. Find a doctor you can relate with, i.e., talk with easily without feeling intimidated.
3. Get copies of all blood tests. You paid for them, you are entitled to them.
4. Keep a daily journal of your symptoms.
5. Write questions and take them to doctors' appointments.
6. Make your doctor explain his or her answers.
7. Ask your doctor to work with you to get your levels to a point where you feel good and enjoy your quality of life.
8. If your doctor refuses to work with you, fire him or her and find another one.
9. Remember, you have a lifelong disease and must take control of your life.
10. Be well.

There's not much to add to Toy Lin's excellent list, except to underscore point number nine: *you* must take control of your life.

LIVING WELL TIP #8:
LISTEN TO AND TRUST YOUR OWN BODY

Listening to and trusting your own body and instincts is an important part of living well. This can be hard if you're not yet diagnosed and are told time and time again "it's in your head," or "it's not your thyroid." After suspecting thyroid disease for many months, but being told by her doctor that there was no reason to even test for hypothyroidism, LuAnn simply *knew* there was something more there. She finally demanded a full thyroid test:

> On Friday evening I received a call from our clinic. It was the doctor on call that night. She said that my bloodwork results had just come in and that she was very worried and needed to get me on some medication immediately. My heart was pounding and I started sobbing on the phone, because someone was saying that, yes, there is actually something wrong with you! She said that my T4 was not even borderline. It was 0.4. And she had never seen a higher TSH, which was 460. But my doctor shocked me when we saw her that Monday. She said, "See, aren't you glad that we checked for thyroid. I kind of thought that that was what was wrong." I told her, "But you said it wasn't thyroid!" She just said "Well, now we know, don't we. Maybe we should have communicated a little better with each other." Oh, was I mad!!! I have never set foot in their clinic again.

Leanne, a thirty-three-year-old thyroid cancer survivor, feels it is important to listen to her body:

> I guess just as important as being informed is being tuned into your own body. I was feeling stressed and short-tempered so I called my doc and asked her to order some bloodwork because I felt I was taking too much Synthroid. That was, in fact, the case. And then a few months later, I told my husband I was still a little high, and the bloodwork verified that. Remember, nobody knows the *normal* you better than you do. Trust yourself.

My doctor is often amazed at how accurate I can be in estimating my TSH levels. I can definitely tell the difference between a TSH of 1.5 versus 4 versus 5.5. If you listen to your body and trust your own instincts, you can probably become quite good at monitoring your own thyroid levels as well.

LIVING WELL TIP #9:
DEVELOP SOME "PERSPECTIVE"—THE ABILITY
TO LOOK BEYOND YOUR THYROID PROBLEM

When you have something like hypothyroidism, which can affect so many aspects of your health, there's a tendency to take it to an extreme. You'll sometimes want to blame everything from your latest toothache to an ingrown toenail on your thyroid.

Ted—an alt.support.thyroid regular—has this to say about having some perspective:

> As you know, in alt.support.thyroid, we can find a reason for *any* symptom to have a root in thyroidland. It is easy to place blame with the thyroid. Many of us get caught up blaming *everything* on our thyroids. I blame my exhaustion on my thyroid. I blame my memory lapses on my thyroid. I blame my bald head on my thyroid. I blame the fact that my washing machine loses socks on my thyroid . . . You would think that the thyroid is *god*.

Ted feels that elevating the thyroid to this level of importance can lead to a sense that tweaking the thyroid dose can cure everything. And if it doesn't, we can end up feeling a profound sense of hopelessness. According to Ted, it's useful to take a step back when therapy seems to fail and look at the various interrelated functions of the body, before assuming that the thyroid is at the core of all the problems. And that's good advice.

I know I have a tendency to assume everything goes wrong because of the thyroid. But sometimes, the several days of unrelenting headache is just a plain old sinus infection. Aches and pains can actually be the flu rather than a developing case of rheumatoid arthritis. And while I assumed I was going to be a standard infertility case and would find it near impossible to get pregnant due to my hypothyroidism, I was pleasantly surprised, becoming pregnant quickly.

The point is, don't assume the worst, and don't always assume it's your thyroid.

LIVING WELL TIP #10:
REDUCE STRESS IN YOUR LIFE

Stress has a major effect on a chronic health concern like hypothyroidism. Stress changes body chemistry and changes your body's need for thyroid hormone, a need that can't always be met on a fixed dosage. Stress also generates brain chemicals that contribute to depression and other disease and make it impossible to heal. When you lower stress, you cause changes in the brain and the immune system that actually increase the ability to fight disease.

Look at the various stressors in your life with an eye toward reducing or eliminating as many as possible. Do you dread weekly housecleaning sessions? Figure out a less stressful way to get them done—perhaps involving your family or hiring a cleaning person. Learn to say "no" to extra obligations and requests from other people. It's one thing to serve as class trip chaperon or take on extra projects at work once in a while. But if you can't say "no," and then find yourself overloaded with other people's hand-me-down projects, focus on learning to say "no" and put your own health and priorities first. "Sorry, I would love to, but I can't possible do that. I have other plans," is a good multipurpose excuse. There's no reason to explain that your other plans include a well-deserved nap or relaxing bath or energizing walk.

Sometimes, reducing the stress in your life may require more dramatic changes, particularly in your job. Bobbi felt it was necessary to switch careers in order to gain more control and less stress in her life:

> I've recently started my own business. I'm cleaning houses and I love it. I used to be a legal/executive secretary stressed out to the max and now I basically work for myself with flexible hours. It's great. I felt like a prisoner and a victim of this disease before. Therapy and a good doctor have made all of the difference in the world! Having an understanding husband, family, and friends have also contributed to my healing process.

Diann is another person who decided to change her job to control her stress:

I have just made a "courageous" choice in life: I have given up my very stressful career of several years, and next week I start clerking at a discount store. I am simplifying my life, paying the credit cards off, eliminating car payments, and just plain getting back to basics. My personal philosophy these days: Life is way too short to struggle past fifty! I grew a fantastic garden this summer. I incorporate all the items in foods I make from "scratch." Our food budget has never looked so good.

Another major source of physical stress is not getting enough sleep. According to a survey released in 1998 by the National Sleep Foundation, one in three people in the United States sleeps for six hours or less per night, substantially less than the recommended eight hours. Sleep is an important way to help restore immune function, and if you used to need seven or eight hours, once hypothyroid, you may need somewhat more on a regular basis to be truly rested. Don't compromise on sleep, or it will definitely add to your stress levels.

In addition to changing careers, learning to assertively say "no," and getting enough sleep, there are many other ways to effectively reduce stress. Exercise, mind-body practices like yoga and T'ai Chi, deep-breathing techniques, meditation, and prayer can all be extremely effective. Some people find that alternative therapies like aromatherapy or listening to relaxation tapes work to reduce stress. It's important to find methods that work for you and to actively practice them, while at the same time removing or reducing those stress factors that you can control.

LIVING WELL TIP #11:
GET TESTED AS OFTEN AS NEEDED

Most of the standard operating manuals for thyroid disease recommend having your thyroid checked once a year—sometimes even once every two years. More frequent testing, however, may be better for you. If you have ongoing problems with symptoms, or unusual symptoms appear, don't wait for your next annual or semi-annual thyroid check. Go in right away.

Renee was glad she had a test earlier than scheduled:

> The doctor I'd been seeing since moving to a new city said every six months would be often enough to check my TSH. In July, my TSH was 2.04 (normal range .2–6). Three months later, I went back and asked for a test because I was exhausted, sleeping, and depressed, mostly. My TSH had shot up to 58 within three months.

Being tested is particularly important to remember when you're going through any hormonal changes, such as post-pregnancy, perimenopause, menopause, or stopping/starting the Pill or hormone replacement therapy.

LIVING WELL TIP #12:
TRY NEW WAYS OF TAKING YOUR MEDICINE

How and when you take your thyroid hormone may have an impact on its effectiveness for you. If things aren't working, and you're taking your thyroid hormone with food, try taking it on an empty stomach. If you take your dose once a day in the morning, try taking it in the evening. If you can split your pill, consider taking some in the morning, some in the evening.

Wayne found that spacing out his dosage was of help in alleviating symptoms:

> I decided I should space out the dosage, taking 0.075 mg when I get up, another 0.075 mg at 3:00 p.m., and 0.050 mg at bedtime. All of a sudden, things seemed to be right. I am awake, alert, but not overly stimulated during the day. When I wake up in the morning I am ready to get out of bed and get going. Since I am an engineer, I did the numbers. I discovered that if I take pills once a day the "ripple"— variation over the day—is very close to 10 percent in the level of T4 (and I assume T3) in the bloodstream. Now, I found out the hard way that a 10 percent change makes all the difference in the world. Taking pills three times a day decreases the ripple to 3 percent, a tolerable number. . . .

Wayne's approach might not work for you, but the key is, when things aren't working, it's time to try something different.

LIVING WELL TIP #13:
MAINTAIN YOUR SENSE OF HUMOR

Doris Lessing wrote: "Laughter is by definition healthy." She was right. A sense of humor goes a long way in dealing with illness.

William F. Fry., M.D., of Stanford University, an expert for the past thirty years on the physiological effects of humor, believes that laughter may actually trigger physical changes that help ease pain. It's thought that laughter causes the brain to release hormones that cause the release of endorphins, the body's natural painkillers. Other scientists have actually documented increased immunity and a reduction in stress hormones during laughter.

All in all, it's clear that humor acts as a critical *vaccine*, protecting your emotional and mental immune system, and can help protect your body from the effects of stress, particularly due to long-term chronic illness. Humor helps bolster your immune system and resilience, and should be a part of your overall program—including nutrition, exercise, rest, emotional satisfaction—for wellness. And beyond the technical, medical reasons, laughter simply does feel good.

I've always tried to incorporate thyroid humor at my thyroid Web site. You might ask, what's so funny about thyroids? It's actually not that hard to find things to laugh about when it comes to thyroid problems, doctors, or HMOs. No one says you need to laugh *about* your thyroid. A funny book, movie, song, or just a good laugh with a friend—all have the same healthful effects.

Find something to make you laugh. . . . laughter *is* the best medicine.

LIVING WELL TIP #14:
MEN—REALIZE THAT YOU'RE NOT ALONE

So many of you men with hypothyroidism feel that you are alone. Dealing with most of the same symptoms that plague women, you also cope with the extra stigma of having what people think of as a "woman's disease." You may feel that no one else understands what you go through.

Bill feels that his bout with hypothyroidism has given him added insight:

> Does it bother me to be a victim of what is known as a woman's disease? Not at all! Women have been an integral part of my life for many years. Having personally experienced the disease, I have a great deal of empathy for "The Sisterhood of the Shattered Butterfly" with all of its unpleasant aspects.

I urge men to join more support groups, or get online and get involved in the online support groups for thyroid disease, where we have many men who regularly participate. You'll be able to share information on some of the unique aspects of hypothyroidism for men, and realize that you are absolutely *not* alone.

LIVING WELL TIP #15:
WOMEN—BE PREPARED FOR
PREGNANCY AND MENOPAUSE

When we're little girls, before we have our first period, our mothers and teachers typically sat down with us and went over one of those cryptic little books about the menstrual cycle and women's anatomy. Often, this is the first and *last* time we actually study and learn about our hormonal cycles—and it's not enough, particularly to get you through pregnancy and menopause.

Pregnancy and menopause can cause hormonal fluctuations for women with hypothyroidism. The shifting hormones can wreak extra havoc on an already unstable endocrine system. To help ride out the ups and downs, I have several key suggestions.

First, get yourself copies of two must-read books. I consider these the absolute basics in any woman's "hormonal library."

• *Screaming to Be Heard: Hormonal Connections Doctors Suspect and Women Ignore,* by Elizabeth Vliet, M.D.

Dr. Vliet's book looks at the impact of hormones on a woman's health. She discusses estrogen, testosterone, perimenopause and full menopause, use of hormone replacement, and the relationships to memory, migraines, fibromyalgia, thyroid problems, and many other women's health issues. It's simply essential reading for every woman.

• *Listening to Your Hormones*, by Gillian Ford

Ford, a specialist on women's hormonal issues, outlines how hormones affect our well-being, and discusses the most common hormonal problems. Ford examines the full range of long- and short-term hormone replacement therapies available today, as well as a host of natural alternatives.

Two, prior to pregnancy, and as you start approaching the age of menopause (keep in mind, you're often likely to go into menopause at about the same time your mother did) be sure to keep detailed records of all your various hormonal levels. It's useful to have baseline levels of estrogen, progesterone, testosterone, and thyroid hormone levels, reflecting a period when you're feeling well. This way, you'll have a target number to work with when you are pregnant, post-partum, and as you become perimenopausal, and ultimately, menopausal. Ask for copies of all bloodwork, and keep charts and copies yourself.

Finally, be sure you're working with a doctor who truly understands women's hormonal medicine. You may need to switch around to find the right doctor. For example, a doctor who doesn't know that pregnant hypothyroid women often need more thyroid hormone is not particularly knowledgeable. A doctor who categorically thinks all menopausal women should be on estrogen is *not* up to date on the latest information in women's medicine.

The right doctor may be a family practice osteopath, or an Ob-Gyn who understands hormonal issues, an endocrinologist, or a practitioner of the newer field of "women's medicine." Whoever it is, make sure he or she is passionate about understanding and staying up to date on all facets of women's hormonal issues, and is open to the full range of options in treating hormonal deficiencies or fluctuations.

LIVING WELL TIP #16:
MAINTAIN A POSITIVE ATTITUDE AND OUTLOOK

I'm the first person to admit that maintaining a positive attitude isn't always easy. And don't let anyone else tell you it is either. Take a person who used to be in perfect health, make them exhausted all the time, add 40 extra pounds, and toss in some fistfuls of hair falling out in big wads, and then show me how many of *them* can maintain a positive attitude! When you add the various health complaints of hypothyroidism, *plus* a tendency toward depression, it's a wonder anyone with hypothyroidism can maintain a positive attitude. But *we* can—and do.

How you stay positive is unique to you. Some people believe in support groups, whether in person, or online. Others find prayer useful. Yet others find aerobic exercise or more mind-body energy exercise such as yoga or T'ai Chi, to be the keys to a sense of well being and positive feelings.

Some days, being positive just means putting one foot in front of the other and moving forward, however you can. Sue has this philosophy when she's not feeling up to par:

> I just put a small goal in front every day and try by the end of the day to get it done . . . even if you start out dusting off three things . . . the next day I try to dust two rooms . . . I can now run the vacuum cleaner and dust!! (Laugh!) I don't let myself get into too much. I expect help and get it . . . if you can't do it, well let it go.

Megan, an upbeat thyroid cancer survivor who exudes positivity herself, has some excellent advice on why a positive attitude is essential:

> It's important to do what makes you happy, stay active, laugh a lot, share your feelings, and keep a positive attitude. Work at this. Tell yourself that for right now, your job is to do whatever you can to have positive things in your life. The biggest choice you have is how to live your life. When you're laying on the couch, unable to even find the energy to go to the kitchen for a piece of bread, make the choice not to let your exhaustion overcome you. Your mind is incredi-

bly powerful, and it will listen if you tell it that you don't want to be depressed or give up. Tell yourself that this exhaustion is temporary, and it doesn't mean you can't still function. You just have to push yourself to keep going. Do small things, then pat yourself on the back that you did them.

Being positive also means being fair about what you expect from yourself. Part of Sue's recovery has been in learning how to move forward positively, but realistically:

My husband, a doctor, understood. He lived with me and had to deal with my lack of energy, fuzziness in concentrating and seeing firsthand how it affected me. He has realized that there is something to this disease. He lets me sleep when I need to and understands the energy spurts and the recovery days. It has impacted my whole family. Maybe replacement is getting back to normal for some people, it wasn't for me. Maybe my doctor thought I was a whiner when all I wanted was to be like I was before. It has been a big adjustment for me and hard to accept that my "normal" was going to have to have a different definition that it did before. I'm more accepting of my limitations. I'm healthy, and live a pretty full, busy life, but I can tell the difference. *Pacing* has become my "word of the day."

Joyce, a quilt artist with hypothyroidism, has found a new philosophy of hope and openness to help her deal with her illness:

Nothing stays constant in life; life is about change and how you handle it. My promise is never to take myself too seriously, to laugh myself through anything and everything, to love, to live every day as though it is my last and to be kind and nonjudgmental. I know as I age, new discoveries will emerge about my disease and perhaps one day, I'll be totally symptom free! For now, I am grateful that I can put a few words together that actually make sense and that I no longer need a padded floor for unscheduled naptime landings. My creativity as a quilt artist has not only returned, it seriously threatens taking over my whole life. I suspect my family and friends are thankful to have the person they vaguely remember back, the one who lives life to the fullest, laughs herself silly and falls to sleep each night with a smile on her face.

The first time I read Joyce's predictions and hope for the future was actually the first time I personally had considered the possibility of a real cure. Every day, it seems, new developments and cures for various diseases are announced, and new medicines or therapies—conventional and alternative—are launched. It's entirely possible that in our lifetimes, we *will* see dramatic improvements in the way hypothyroidism is treated, especially if we patients work together to insist on this progress. And pondering those thoughts *definitely* gives me a positive attitude.

LIVING WELL TIP #17:
AIM TO BE A SUCCESS STORY

Ultimately, living well with hypothyroidism means deciding that you are going to be a person who voyages through life, rising above the hypothyroidism. You may ultimately learn to live with it, work around it, even reverse or cure it, but somehow, you will live well. Susan has found her own answer to living well:

> I had obvious thyroid symptoms for years but "normal" TSH that kept creeping up: 2.5, 3.5. 5.2, etc. I was the one who did the research and insisted on an antibody test when my throat felt swollen in the thyroid area. This was with the horrible primary doc who used to just shrug and dismiss all my inquiries. I have new docs for myself now who are much more respectful. My new primary started me on thyroid hormone replacement when I asked to be retested at her lab and my TSH was 7.2 and antibodies sky high. She set me up with a decent endo who also listens pretty well. I'm hanging in at 2.5 TSH and although I may be able to do better, I feel pretty good in comparison to before, and am down 14 pounds!

Pam is excited to be finally back on track with her life and health:

Right now, I feel that I am feeling the best I have for twenty years. My ability to think, concentrate, and express myself has much improved due to thyroid meds and hormone replacement therapy. You have to advocate for yourself (or be lucky enough to find a doctor who really understands thyroid). Low thyroid is so subtle in the way it takes away your life—slowly, slowly, slowly taking away your health, your thinking abilities, and due to tiredness, your relationships, your recreational activities. It's amazing to me to wake up out of this fog, and now to have so far to go to catch up and gain my life back. For the first time in years, I feel good enough to want to exercise!

Suzanne has had to redefine somewhat her expectations and, in doing so, has learned how to live well.

I feel great actually, lots of energy most of the time. Now and then a few symptoms will be noticeable but I don't let them keep me down. I'm not sure about other thyroid sufferers, endos or doctors, but to be told that you are now in your forties and things are just the way they are and get used to it—I don't agree. Sure, some things aren't going to be quite the same but other things can be dealt with and between the doctor and the patient a happy medium should be able to be met.

As you embark on your own journey toward living well with hypothyroidism, I have two thoughts. First, "carpe diem," as they say in Latin—"seize the day!" Second, as my friend Ted from alt.-support.thyroid says: "Carpe Thyroidiem! Seize the Thyroid . . . Wrestle it to the Ground if You Have To!"

As we say online—"LOL!"—laugh out loud!

May you always live well.

Epilogue:
Critical Hypothyroidism Issues
for the Twenty-First Century

The best way to predict the future is to invent it.
ALAN KAY

During the first half of the twentieth century hypothyroidism was diagnosed by a variety of different tests and criteria. It was treated with natural thyroid hormone. The second half of the twentieth century will be remembered for the rise—and subsequent dominance—of the TSH test and levothyroxine.

What will the next century bring us in terms of hypothyroidism treatment? Hopefully, books like this will be just the beginning of patient-directed efforts to gain a greater voice in thyroid treatment. Together, we can speak out about the need for long-overdue research and breakthroughs in hypothyroidism diagnosis and treatment. At the same time, we need to energize the nearly nonexistent search for ways to prevent, reverse, or even cure some forms of hypothyroidism.

As we begin the twenty-first century, you—whether you are a thyroid patient, friend, or family member of a thyroid patient, or healthcare practitioner—have a *critical* role in ensuring that diagnosis and treatment for hypothyroidism does not remain static for the next fifty or 100 years. Start by speaking out and taking an active role in some of the following important issues of hypothyroidism in the twenty-first century.

"NORMAL" TSH LEVELS NEED TO BE STUDIED

The current TSH levels used by laboratories to define the "normal" range of thyroid function, and the use of the TSH test as a primary means of diagnosis need to be significantly reevaluated. The .5 to 5.5 "normal" range for thyroid function does not give enough information for diagnosis anymore. Research reported in the *British Medical Journal* found that TSH levels above 2 are likely not normal and instead include people at high risk to develop thyroid disease. This means that the real "normal" range is probably far narrower and more concentrated at the lower end.

New studies need to be conducted to look at this issue comprehensively, evaluating the true normal range for a population of individuals who have *no thyroid antibodies* and who do not *ever* go on to develop thyroid disease in their lifetimes.

In addition to looking at new definitions of the normal range, quality of life research needs to be conducted that defines narrower target TSH ranges where symptoms are minimized or eliminated, without serious longterm health dangers. This *must* take into account patients' reports of symptoms, quality of life, energy, fatigue, weight gain, and all the other symptoms that frequently continue in "treated" hypothyroidism. It's not enough to determine one target range for all adults of all ages. These ranges must look at optimal TSH levels specific to a variety of different population groups and circumstances, including:

* Infants
* Adolescent Boys
* Adult Men
* Senior Men
* Adolescent, Premenstrual Girls
* Women in Different Hormonal States, i.e., Menstruating, Pregnant, Perimenopausal, Menopausal, and Postmenopausal

Other questions need to be studied, including:

* How thyroid hormone requirements in a woman change during the menstrual cycle, how this can be reproduced with a better

form of thyroid hormone delivery, i.e., a patch, or a daily pill with changing dosage based on the menstrual cycle.

- How TSH fluctuates during the day, and whether it warrants administering thyroid hormone by other means, such as different dosages split throughout the day or via time-released pills, for optimum results and reduction of symptoms.
- More in-depth understanding of how to prescribe thyroid hormone based on the seasonal fluctuations that are known to occur in TSH levels and the body's inhibited ability to convert T4 to T3 during cold weather.
- If and how major physical stress, disease, surgery, pregnancy, and breastfeeding warrant specific or planned modifications in dosage to meet the body's thyroid hormone requirements, and what the implications are for optimal treatment.

BIG PROFITS MEAN LITTLE INCENTIVE FOR INFORMATION OR RESEARCH

Each thyroid patient spends—whether directly or via medical coverage—several hundred dollars a year at least on thyroid hormone replacement, plus additional costs for periodic TSH tests and doctor visits related to the hypothyroidism. Thyroid disease and its treatment, therefore, represent a highly profitable arena for some drug manufacturers, laboratories, and doctors. It's absolutely essential that thyroid patients—as well as lawmakers and the media—become far more aware of the negative influence that the "profitability" of hypothyroidism has on our current health, the state of thyroid research, and the implications for the health and welfare of our children and future generations.

For most of the 1990s, Synthroid, the top-selling brand of levothyroxine, was the *third most prescribed medicine in the U.S.* This means that brands of levothyroxine, including Synthroid—which alone is estimated to control 85 percent of the total market for levothyroxine—are major moneymakers in the U.S. and around the world.

The fact that the business of levothyroxine is so lucrative has many downsides for you as a thyroid patient First, there is no real incentive for manufacturers to inform you about alternatives to levothyroxine, options that might, in fact, be better able to help resolve your symptoms. Many of the "educational" pamphlets about hypothyroidism handed out to patients in doctors' offices are thinly disguised marketing brochures, provided free to doctors by the pharmaceutical companies that manufacture levothyroxine. This information presents only one side of the hypothyroidism story that, of course, favors products sold by the brochure's sponsor.

Second, maintaining, and even gaining, market share is a key mission of most pharmaceutical manufacturers. To that end, a tremendous amount of time and money is spent conducting aggressive marketing and sales efforts to introduce even first-year medical students to their drugs. There's also ongoing marketing efforts designed to steer practicing doctors away from products sold by competitors, even though those competitors may sell similar or alternative drugs that are equally effective, safe, and FDA-approved. This heavy marketing also means that the primary, and sometimes sole, source of information about thyroid drugs for many doctors may be the pharmaceutical companies selling those drugs.

Third, many professional endocrinological organizations rely on pharmaceutical company funding, and their members benefit from a variety of private and institutional research grant funding. These organizations and their members, therefore, are far less likely to do or say anything that isn't in the interests of the drug companies who hold the purse strings. So there is a self-perpetuating insularity and a built-in resistance to anything new or to alternatives that challenge the dominance of the predominant thyroid drugs.

Fourth, much like the professional organizations, most of the major patient service organizations, also primarily run by doctors, rely on pharmaceutical company funding to a varying extent. These organizations publicly claim to represent patients but are noticeably absent on key patient issues that might involve criticism of drug companies. This potential conflict of interest has serious and long-term implications for patients and our wellness.

Fifth, since a substantial part of research into thyroid disease is funded by major manufacturers of thyroid drugs, it is not likely that any meaningful research will be conducted that could truly *improve the quality of life* of people with hypothyroidism. Manufacturers are not likely to fund research into prevention of hypothyroidism, search for real cures for hypothyroidism (that would replace lifelong treatment with levothyroxine), explore alternative drugs or therapies that might have better results for some people, or study the side effects of their levothyroxine products. This is an important point. *There is no incentive for manufacturers to research cures because there is no reason to fund research that might result in reduced sales of levothyroxine, the drug they profit from selling in the first place.*

Nearly all mainstream research on drugs involves the manufacturers in some way. According to an investigation by the *New England Journal of Medicine,* 96 percent of the doctors, scientists, and researchers who write articles supporting particular drugs or therapies receive some financial benefit from the pharmaceutical companies that make the drugs.

This influence makes it all the more important for patients to take it upon themselves to get more information about their hypothyroidism. You can't assume that you will get complete, balanced, and unbiased information from patient brochures, pharmaceutical company-sponsored informational sessions, or doctors who may be biased due to sponsorships, research funding, or their medical education.

THE DOMINANCE OF SYNTHROID

Many people incorrectly use the term "Synthroid" as a generic term for all thyroid medication, reflecting the company's predominance in the thyroid hormone market. This predominance is the result of years of effort, and millions of dollars in support for professional and patient groups, sponsorship of public awareness campaigns, and marketing and advertising efforts. While the company that manufacturers Synthroid does make some positive contributions to thyroid awareness, there are also things you should know about the company that has such an influence on hypothyroidism treatment.

To help consolidate its marketing position in the 1980s, Boots Pharmaceuticals, Synthroid's manufacturer at the time, commissioned and funded a study to demonstrate that Synthroid was superior to its competitors. They were trying to justify the company's practice of charging up to twice the price of competitive products. Unfortunately, study results did not prove that Synthroid was superior. They found that Synthroid was bioequivalent to other brand names of levothyroxine. Instead of publishing the research, the company questioned the research they themselves commissioned, and, over the author's objections, the research was not published. After seven years, in April 1997, the study was finally published over the company's objections in the *Journal of the American Medical Association*.

In May 1997, an $8.5 billion class action lawsuit against the manufacturer of Synthroid, Knoll Pharmaceuticals and parent company BASF, was filed. The lawsuit charged that patients should be compensated for overpaying for Synthroid for up to seven years—the period between when the study was completed and its publication—because the product was not superior to its competitors.

In August 1997, just several months later, Knoll agreed to a proposed settlement of the class action lawsuit. By all estimates, the announcement of a settlement seemed a lightening-fast resolution of a process that typically takes years. It also seemed to benefit primarily the manufacturer, as under the proposed program, each patient would receive an average of less than $19. This $19 was just a fraction of estimated overpayment in the range of $40 to $60 per year—or $264 to $408—for each patient who was on Synthroid the full six-and-one-half years that results were not published.

The $135 million settlement cap represented only a tiny fraction of what the many millions of patients taking Synthroid likely overpaid. It seemed that besides the manufacturer, Knoll Pharmaceuticals, the only people who would truly benefit from the settlement were the class action law firms involved in this unusually rapid class action settlement, who would earn their millions of dollars in fees before patients were even paid.

That spring and summer of 1997, I contacted the main organization for thyroid patients in the U.S., the Thyroid Foundation of America. In addition, I contacted the American Medical Women's Association, sponsors of the major "GlandCentral" thyroid awareness advertising and outreach campaign, which is funded by Knoll

Pharmaceutical, Synthroid's manufacturer. I asked these organizations to publicly comment on what appeared to be a rush to settlement that did not benefit thyroid patients or compensate them in any way for the amount of money overpaid for Synthroid. In particular, I expected the Thyroid Foundation of America to be appalled that patients, their paying members, had overpaid in the hundreds of dollars and were being mistreated by such a paltry settlement.

Unfortunately, neither organization—with their supposed missions to educate, support, and serve as advocates for thyroid patients—said they felt it was at all within their purview to publicly address this concern.

A fairness hearing in March 1998 allowed people dissatisfied with the proposed settlement payoff to exclude themselves from the class action lawsuit, and a number of people exercised this option. In August 1998, the federal judge blocked the proposed $98 million settlement. While Knoll believed the settlement was fair, consumer groups, attorneys generals, and others, including me, had protested that the deal was compensating law firms millions of dollars and represented many millions less than the estimated $500 million to $1.5 billion Knoll might be liable for in a fair settlement. The *Wall Street Journal* even reported that the judge felt that the amount of fees sought suggested the possibility that the settlement is "driven by fees."

In December 1998, the judge held a status conference in this litigation and scheduled further proceedings in the litigation through October 1999. No trial date has yet been set. As this book goes to press, it appears that no money will be paid to any class members unless and until a class is certified by the court and the class obtains a final judgment in its favor after trial, or a further settlement is agreed upon and approved by the court. The holdup is probably even worse for patients than the settlement. Before, the company had to pay less than $20 a person. While the lawsuit drags on, they don't have to pay patients anything.

Instead of waiting around for a settlement that may never happen, join the Thyroid Foundation of America, pay your dues, and speak up loud and often, and insist that they represent you, *not* the pharmaceutical company interests that provide financial support. Ask the questions that no one wants to answer and keep insisting that the thyroid patient organizations answer them if they want to keep you as a member. Ask your doctor if he or she is receiving funding, grants, freebies, perks, or anything else of material value from the pharmaceutical manufacturers. And if so, ask if he or she can honestly be impartial about prescribed drugs.

Your doctors, the nation's researchers, and *our* patient organizations cannot serve two masters—the patient *and* the pharmaceutical companies. Right now, there appear to be serious questions about who is being served. If we want this to change, every single one of us needs to speak up about the big business of hypothyroidism, or we're putting our health and lives in the hands of companies and doctors who don't see us as patients but, instead, as dollar signs.

COST DIFFERENTIALS

Before you fill your prescription, it's important to know that the brand of thyroid hormone your doctor prescribes can mean a difference of hundreds of dollars a year, even though there is no difference in the drugs themselves. The brand name levothyroxine drugs—such as Levoxyl, Levothroid, and Synthroid—have been proven to be bioequivalent, meaning they are considered interchangeable. So a 50 microgram tablet of Synthroid is basically the same as a 50 microgram tablet of Levoxyl, and so on. The brand you're prescribed has to do your doctor's preferences and susceptibility to the marketing of manufacturers, not the quality or consistency of the prescribed drug.

Before you have a prescription filled, you might want to check with the pharmacy to compare prices of the top thyroid drugs. Synthroid, for example, is often twice the cost of Levoxyl per month. In May 1999, for example, at one pharmacy, a monthly prescription of .2 dosage Synthroid costs $19.20 versus $10.40 for Levoxyl, an $8.80 per month difference that translates to more than $100 per year.

When the consumer is paying, the price of Synthroid is still substantially more than its competitors at most drugstores. A 1999 House Government Reform and Oversight Committee found that the monthly retail cost of Synthroid to seniors paying out of pocket for the drug was $27.05, 1,446 percent more than the $1.75 paid by favored group purchasers such as HMOs.

You can fight back. If your doctor prescribes Synthroid, you could ask him or her about one of the less expensive—but equally effective, safe, and reliable—brand name, not generic—levothyroxine products, like Levoxyl, or Levothroid. Is there a reason to pay a high price when equivalent, less expensive brand name products will work just as well?

REAL REGULATION AND ASSESSMENT OF LEVOTHYROXINE

All prescription drugs have gone through the same testing and approval process, right? Not so for levothyroxine drugs. Synthroid, the first levothyroxine product, never went through formal testing when it was introduced in the 1950s. It was essentially "grandfathered in" as equivalent to natural thyroid hormone products. Because it never went through the application and approval process, there is no trial data on Synthroid or levothyroxine to prove the claims that it is superior to the natural thyroid drugs used in the first half of the century. There is also little formal collection of information on side effects, minor and serious. Levothyroxine needs to be regulated—truly, honestly, formally, and fully regulated.

In 1997, the FDA reported that levothyroxine drugs are officially classified as "new" drugs and will need to go through the new drug application process. This decision was due to stability and potency problems that came to light. They found that often levothyroxine sodium drugs do not remain potent through their expiration dates, and tablets of the same dosage strength from the same manufacturer have been found to vary in potency from lot to lot in the amount of active ingredient present. The *Federal Register* wrote: "no currently marketed orally administered levothyroxine sodium product has been shown to demonstrate consistent potency and stability. . . ."

In order to continue marketing these drugs, manufacturers needed to submit a new drug application with documented evidence that each company's product is safe, effective, and manufactured in a way to ensure consistent potency. Because the drug is necessary to millions of Americans, the FDA will allow manufacturers to continue to market these products without approvals until August 14, 2000, in order to give companies enough time to conduct the various research studies and to submit their NDAs.

One benefit of this process is that additional information will become available about the side effects of levothyroxine. Most side effects from levothyroxine are not understood, or even known, because manufacturers have been required to report only unexpected and serious side effects of these drugs.

Another benefit may be better efforts at consistency. Since the initiation of these products, almost every manufacturer of orally administered levothyroxine sodium products, including Synthroid, has regularly reported recalls due to potency or stability problems. In some cases, problems result from the fact that levothyroxine potency is unstable after continued exposure to light, heat, air, and humidity. Just since 1991, there have been more than ten recalls of levothyroxine tablets involving 150 lots and more than 100 million tablets. In most cases, the recalls were initiated because tablets were found to be subpotent or because their levothyroxine tablets lose potency before their expiration dates, or occasionally, because a product was found to be too potent.

Problems also stem from formulation changes. Because these products were never required to pass the new drug application process, manufacturers have not had to file for FDA approval each time they reformulate their levothyroxine products. Manufacturers have changed inactive ingredients, changed the physical form of coloring agents and other product aspects, resulting in significant changes in potency, in some cases increasing or decreasing potency, *by as much as 30 percent.* As a result, in some cases, people on the same dosage for years became toxic on what was *sold* as the same dose. According to the FDA, there is evidence that manufacturers continue to make these sorts of formulation changes that affect potency.

While every batch of levothyroxine is not necessarily a problem of potency, over time, the erratic potency of these drugs can have a number of implications for those of us on longterm thyroid hormone replacement. You and your doctor may find it difficult to stabilize you at your optimal TSH level on the same dose of the same drug, if pills themselves vary in dosage, or from batch to batch potency varies. You may suffer symptoms of hypothyroidism or hyperthyroidism when you are under- or over-medicated.

Until the new drug application process is completed, pay particular attention to symptoms that develop after refilling a prescription or changing pharmacies or brands, and be sure to discuss them with your doctor.

EFFECTIVENESS OF LEVOTHYROXINE VERSUS THE USE OF T3

Once and for all, the question of whether some, or maybe all, people with hypothyroidism would have substantial improvements in health with the addition of T3 to their thyroid hormone therapy must be decided to even the satisfaction of the most conventional, close-minded doctors.

There's no question that T3 is a critical part of adequate thyroid hormone replacement for some people. But the use of T3 is, for the most part, still relegated to "alternative" treatment and is not part of thyroid replacement therapy for most hypothyroid patients in the U.S. Most of the conventional medical authorities advocate the use of brand name levothyroxine/synthetic T4 alone as treatment for hypothyroidism. These doctors do not recommend the addition of T3 to the regimen, whether it comes from synthetic T3 drugs like Cytomel, or the combination synthetic T4/T3 drug Thyrolar, or the natural thyroid hormone replacement drugs like Armour.

These practices persist despite the research study, reported in February 1999 in the *New England Journal of Medicine*, discussed in chapter 8. That study demonstrated a clear physical, cognitive, and psychological benefit to most patients taking some T3 along with their T4 drug. The *New England Journal of Medicine* study—though it will continue to be attacked because it threatens the highly profitable TSH testing and levothyroxine market—showed that T3 offered a clear benefit to a majority of patients.

In addition to the *New England Journal of Medicine* article, there is other research that suggests that T3 may work better for some people. Research reported in *Obstetrics and Gynecology* in 1990 found that patients on levothyroxine needed additional dosage to maintain a normal TSH level during pregnancy. In addition, whether pregnant or not, patients treated with levothyroxine only showed a lower T3 to T4 ratio, a ratio related to peripheral conversion of T4 to T3, than the normal population. The ratio decreased even more during pregnancy, and so relative deficiency of T3 during pregnancy was suspected in levothyroxine-treated patients. In contrast, patients who were on natural desiccated thyroid that includes T3 (i.e., Armour) *did not require any change in dosage, as their TSH did not change during pregnancy, nor was their T3 to T4 ratio out of balance.*

Thyroid drugs with T3 are safe, effective, and FDA-approved. In the case of natural thyroid hormone like Armour, we're talking about a product that was used almost exclusively and safely the entire first half of the century. Dozens of seniors have contacted me saying that their doctors took them off Armour after twenty or thirty years or more, and only *then* did symptoms begin to plague them after years of good health on Armour. Many of the oldtime doctors *still* prefer Armour because they simply can't get satisfying results with levothyroxine alone.

When you look at all these factors, the implications are clear. All doctors, not just alternative practitioners, should seriously consider the possible benefits of adding T3 for patients who have unrelieved symptoms and health complaints related to their hypothyroidism. Anything less is not providing the best possible care for patients.

The message here is that not only do rational doctors need to consider the use of T3 for patients, but T3 should also be intensively researched. Questions need to be answered, such as: How much T3 does the body need? What problems or conditions might impede T4 to T3 transformation? Are there certain situations or conditions where patients would *definitely* do better with the addition of T3?

More research is also needed on the role of Reverse T3. Reverse T3 refers to the process by which the body converts T4, not to T3, but to an inactive form, Reverse T3, during times of physical stress. A 1977 report in the *Journal of Clinical Endocrinology and Metabolism* found that both pregnancy and estrogen administration were associated with increases in Reverse T3 concentrations, for example. Does this increase in Reverse T3 during periods of hormonal upheaval explain why women with hypothyroidism tend to suffer greater fluctuations and worsening of symptoms after pregnancy, or during menopause, or after starting the Pill or hormone replacement therapy? This is something that deserves serious study by impartial researchers.

When it comes to the T3 issue, the *New England Journal of Medicine* article provided evidence that what patients had been saying for years—and what had until then been summarily dismissed by most doctors—is likely. It is now time to explore more fully the role of T3 in proper treatment for hypothyroidism.

BETTER SCREENING FOR AND DIAGNOSIS OF HYPOTHYROIDISM

A study presented at the 1997 annual meeting of the American Thyroid Association looked at a large population sample, 25,862 study participants, and found 2,456 people who had elevated TSH levels, indicative of some degree of thyroid gland failure and resulting hypothyroidism. Of those people, 2,198 people were not receiving thyroid medication. This was the largest study ever conducted to examine the prevalence of thyroid disease, and it found that 11.7 percent of the study participants had abnormal thyroid function, yet only one percent of the total population was receiving treatment.

Why aren't these people being diagnosed and treated for their hypothyroidism? As we've seen before, some of them don't even mention their symptoms to doctors, and aren't aware that what they're going through isn't simply aging, or fatigue, or the results of weight gain, or other excuses. Others have discussed their symptoms, but are ignored or patronized by physicians who can't be bothered to run a TSH test, or who aren't enough familiar with the symptoms of hypothyroidism to suspect the problem.

Doctors need to become vastly more aware of the prevalence of thyroid disease. They need to learn to recognize the many possible symptoms and know to test for thyroid problems when any one of the common symptoms appears, and who is most at risk for developing the condition. Cameron, a woman in her twenties, wrote to me and said that she'd had to go to a second doctor for diagnosis, after she asked for a thyroid test and was told by her gynecologist that hypothyroidism "didn't affect younger women, only women after menopause." This is, of course, completely wrong.

In my opinion, when it comes to testing, every time a woman gets an annual gynecological exam she should also have a thyroid function test, especially after pregnancy and as she nears menopause. This screening and testing should be included in regular preventive checkups, covered by insurance. The medical, psychiatric, and psychological communities should make thyroid testing standard before prescribing any antidepressants. And thyroid tests should be part of routine blood work for physicals and medical evaluation for men and women of all ages.

THE DANGERS OF UNDERTREATMENT OR NONTREATMENT

Recent studies have suggested that thyroid levels above 2 are actually more representative of a failing, rather than a healthy, thyroid. These studies mean that there's a potential epidemic of undertreated and misdiagnosed hypothyroidism. Millions of people with "treated" hypothyroidism may actually be *undertreated*, and millions of people with hypothyroidism are going undiagnosed and left untreated.

The undertreatment issue is one most patients know well. A study presented at the 1997 American Thyroid Association meeting found that of those taking medication for both elevated- and low-thyroid hormone levels, an amazing 40 percent still had an abnormal TSH level. Their TSH levels were not being properly controlled.

There is no doubt that untreated or undertreated hypothyroidism has a number of health risks, including:

- cardiovascular disease
- high cholesterol levels
- weight gain and obesity
- depression
- reduced physical activity
- danger during pregnancy to both mother and baby

There is even some scientific evidence that in the long term, higher TSH levels can increase the risk of thyroid cancer.

A study presented at the American Thyroid Association meeting confirmed that an underactive thyroid can result in high cholesterol levels. Gay Canaris, M.D., of the University of Nebraska Medical Center and lead author of the study, has said:

> Each year, almost two million people suffer a heart attack or stroke. The better we can help people control their thyroid condition, the better we can help them manage or even bring down their cholesterol levels, a major risk factor to coronary artery complications.

The primary argument doctors make against keeping the TSH level in the low end of the range is the danger of osteoporosis, which is discussed next. But definitive research needs to be conducted to weigh the dangers associated with undertreatment of hypothyroidism versus doses that maintain low normal TSH levels.

THE REAL RISK OF OSTEOPOROSIS

Some studies demonstrate that doses of levothyroxine that suppress thyroid function—essentially causing hyperthyroidism, or extremely low TSH levels—can be a risk factor for osteoporosis. Just as many other major studies, however, found no significant reduction in bone mass in people with a suppressed TSH, hence no increased risk of osteoporosis. These studies looked at osteoporosis in patients who had suppressed TSH levels. Suppressed levels are typically *below* the .3 to .7 considered to be the low end of the *normal* range at many U.S. labs.

While the research is contradictory, some doctors have only

heard the findings that showed very low TSH levels can increase osteoporosis risk. These doctors decide that if a very low TSH level poses a risk, then why not keep people at higher levels, and thereby avoid the risk? Hence, the current penchant on the part of some doctors to get patients to high-normal TSH levels and declare the patients fully euthyroid. These patients then walk around feeling unwell, being told it's not their thyroid, with the doctor refusing to prescribe a higher dose of thyroid hormone.

This fear of the low end of the normal range also completely ignores the many studies that clearly demonstrate that functional hypothyroidism, which can take place in the normal range for some people, clearly has a detrimental impact on health. Affected areas include cholesterol levels, heart disease, and many other major health concerns that may be far more serious than a possible—and as yet not definitively proven—risk of osteoporosis.

Comprehensive and definitive research needs to be conducted to decide once and for all whether suppressed, low-normal, or even *mid-normal* TSH levels are "dangerous" or increase the risk of osteoporosis. This risk also needs to be assessed in comparison to the many other health risks—including the very real risk of heart disease, America's number one killer—that are associated with higher TSH levels or physiologic hypothyroidism.

THE NEED FOR RESEARCH INTO ALTERNATIVE THERAPIES

Conventional medicine is wedded to the treatment of the condition—levothyroxine to replace the missing thyroid hormone. But for people who still have a thyroid capable of functioning, alternative medicine offers the tantalizing possibility of returning the thyroid to normal, or the potential to even prevent, slow, stop, and even reverse some forms of hypothyroidism and thyroid disease. And barring complete "cures," alternative medicine also offers potentially effective options for treatment of unresolved symptoms, such as fatigue and weight gain.

It is clear that some of the therapies for hypothyroidism—such as Chinese medicine, acupuncture, osteopathy, herbs, nutrition/supplements, yoga, and homeopathy, among other treatments—can help hypothyroidism and its symptoms. Unfortunately, each effective alternative treatment rarely comes with a definitive medical journal article proving its effectiveness or an easy-to-follow treatment protocol. Instead, most of what is known and practiced is literally in the heads of individual practitioners, or is part of an alternative system's accepted body of knowledge, such as in traditional Chinese Medicine.

Self-guided research seems to be the norm. For example, Susan Osborne, an osteopathic physician in Floyd, Virginia, is studying antibody levels in her patients. Through repeated testing of patients with autoimmune hypothyroidism, Dr. Osborne has found that many people have higher antibody levels when they eat larger quantities of refined sugar products.

Ayurvedic doctors are finding that they can effectively treat some cases of hypothyroidism using the ayurvedic herbal remedy guggul, which has the added benefit of substantially lowering cholesterol levels and blood fats. Dr. Osborne's discovery and the developments in ayurvedic medicine are just a few of the sort of exciting, groundbreaking alternative treatments that should be the focus of intensive interest by medical practitioners.

Unfortunately, there is strong resistance to alternative medicine and therapies. This resistance stems from the mainstream healthcare industry's economic interest to prevent consumer health dollars from flowing to alternative practitioners and remedies. But at the same time, the resistance also stems from the rigid adherence to mainstream-style, peer-reviewed "research" that drives conventional medical knowledge. Unfortunately, since few companies are likely to profit from rigorous testing of products like guggul or from dietary approaches to lowering antibody levels, and since the profile for hypothyroidism is not high, the kind of research that satisfies the mainstream medical establishment isn't likely to occur. It's inexplicable, for example, that among all the alternative research projects currently funded by the National Institutes of Health, something as common as hypothyroidism is not well represented.

We patients need to continue to ask that this sort of research take a higher priority with patient organizations and federally funded programs.

THE THYROID, ESTROGEN, PROGESTERONE CONNECTION

The relationship between thyroid, estrogen, and progesterone is one that begs for additional study and research. It's known that the thyroid contains receptors for estrogen, and that estrogen imbalances can inhibit proper thyroid hormone secretion. Excessive estrogen, a shortage of progesterone, or a combination of both problems may lead to a condition known as estrogen dominance. The symptoms of estrogen dominance are very similar to side effects and symptoms of hypothyroidism, and, in fact, hypothyroidism is sometimes considered a symptom of estrogen dominance.

According to menopause educator and thyroid patient Pat Rackowski:

> Imbalances of thyroid hormones T3 and T4, combined with imbalances of estrogen and progesterone, can produce many different consequences in the areas of mood, temperature regulation, fluid retention, and energy. One critical area that cries out for extensive research is the relationship between the thyroid and the two key female hormones, estrogen and progesterone.

Some women have found that receiving progesterone treatment (via natural progesterone, not synthetic progestins) balances out estrogen dominance and can return slight hypothyroidism to normal levels, or make thyroid hormone replacement therapy more effective and eliminate unrelieved symptoms. This is commonly a problem during periods when estrogen dominance can take place naturally, such as after pregnancy, during perimenopause and menopause, or after beginning hormone replacement therapy or birth control pills.

Since it's known that excess estrogen can be a key factor in many autoimmune diseases, this hormonal interdependence, thyroid disease, and the relationship to autoimmunity are all fertile subjects for research.

IODINE DEFICIENCY AND THYROID DISEASE

As mentioned earlier, a deficiency of iodine is one of the basic causes of hypothyroidism and goiter in countries where there isn't sufficient iodine. Earlier in this century, iodized salt was thought to have almost wiped out iodine deficiency in the U.S. In recent years, there's been a strong difference of opinion between some alternative practitioners and herbalists, who recommend iodine or kelp supplements for hypothyroidism, and other doctors, who argue that iodine is not only not needed, but can worsen thyroid problems, particularly autoimmune conditions.

There is, however, a new finding that has a major impact on the iodine/no-iodine issue: iodine deficiency is back in the U.S. The October 1998 issue of the *Journal of Clinical Endocrinology and Metabolism* reported that in the last twenty years, the percentage of Americans with low intake of iodine has more than quadrupled. Researchers indicated that this trend might necessitate concerted efforts to increase iodine levels in people at risk of deficiency. The first National Health and Nutrition Examination Survey (NHANES I), which took place from 1971 to 1974, found that just 2.6 percent of U.S. citizens had iodine deficiency. The followup NHANES III survey, conducted from 1988 to 1994, found that 11.7 percent are iodine deficient. Of particular concern is the fact that the percentage of iodine-deficient pregnant women has increased from 1 percent in 1974 to 7 percent in 1994. Iodine deficiency during pregnancy is particularly dangerous to a growing baby.

Researchers do not have an explanation for this change, though they suspect that reduced salt in the diet, plus a reduction in the use of iodine as a food ingredient, may be responsible. The reasons for this increasing deficiency need to be studied, and those at risk of iodine deficiency in the U.S. need to be made more aware of this potential risk for hypothyroidism.

SOY FORMULAS AND SOY FOODS—
A THYROID DANGER

Dr. Mike Fitzpatrick is an environmental scientist and phytoestrogen researcher who has extensively researched the issue of soy formulas, and the impact of soy consumption on thyroid function. Dr. Fitzpatrick introduced me to a little-known fact that can have substantial impact on people with hypothyroidism and the population in general: overconsumption of soy products has the potential to impair thyroid function.

Dr. Fitzpatrick is so concerned that he is calling for soy formula manufacturers to remove the isoflavones, agents that are most active against the thyroid, from their products.

According to Dr. Fitzpatrick, since the late 1950s, it has been known that soy formulas contain antithyroid agents. Cases of goiter were reported in soy-formula-fed infants until manufacturers added more iodine to their products. The antithyroid agents in soy have recently been identified as what are known as *isoflavones*. Soy is a rich source of isoflavones, and Dr. Fitzpatrick found that infants fed soy infant formulas receive high daily doses of these compounds.

The isoflavones belong to the flavonoid chemical family, and flavonoids are considered endocrine disruptors—plants that act as hormones, disrupting the endocrine system. Flavonoids are, in particular, well-known antithyroid agents. (The grain millet, for example, contains high levels of flavonoids and is commonly known as problematic for those with low thyroid function.) Flavonoids typically act against the thyroid by inhibition of thyroid peroxidase (TPO), which disturbs proper thyroid function. Isoflavones are no exception, and they are potent inhibitors of TPO.

A preliminary study found a significant association between feeding soy formulas and the development of autoimmune thyroid disease in infants. One study found that the frequency of feedings with soy-based milk formulas in early life was noticeably higher in children with autoimmune thyroid disease. Thyroid problems were almost triple in those soy-formula-fed children compared to their siblings and healthy unrelated children. Dr. Fitzpatrick raises another major concern for infants on soy formula:

> Long-term feeding of soy formulas will result in persistent inhibition of TPO and a continual tendency toward elevated TSH levels. This state is associated with the induction of thyroid cancer in laboratory animals.

In other words, infants who are exposed to high concentrations of isoflavones long-term, such as that found in a diet of primarily soy formula, may face a risk of becoming hypothyroid, and even face an increased chance of developing thyroid cancer.

There are also concerns for adult consumption of soy products. One U.K. study involving premenopausal women gave 60 grams of soy protein per day for one month. This was found to disrupt the menstrual cycle, with the effects of the isoflavones continuing for a full three months after soy in the diet was stopped. Another study found that intake of soy over a long period causes enlargement of the thyroid and suppresses thyroid function. Isoflavones are also known to modify fertility and change sex hormone status and to have serious health effects—including infertility, thyroid disease, or liver disease—on a number of mammals.

Next Steps?

According to Dr. Fitzpatrick, the soy industry has known about the goitrogenic and estrogenic effects of soy for more than sixty years. But in that time, far too little has been done to truly address these concerns, particularly in the United States, where the health benefits of soy are being extensively marketed, particularly to menopausal women and women at risk of breast cancer.

In July 1996, the British Department of Health issued a warning that the phytoestrogens found in soy-based infant formulas could adversely affect infant health. The warning was clear, indicating that soy formula should only be given to babies on the advice of a health professional. They advised that babies who cannot be breastfed or who have allergies to other formulas be given alternatives to soy-based formulas. That same year, the British government's Food Advisory Committee also asked companies to investigate the removal of soy isoflavones from soy-based infant formulas. It is technically possible to remove the actual isoflavones from soy-based infant formulas, and some companies have developed test versions of these products, but they are not readily available for consumers. It appears, however, that most formula manufacturers do not plan to modify their manufacturing process to permanently remove the isoflavones, and thereby reduce the risk.

Infants are particularly vulnerable when exposed to endocrine disruptors. Because infants fed soy formula are receiving the highest exposure to isoflavones, they are at risk of chronic thyroid problems. Long-term research on this unplanned "test group" of infants, who subsisted solely on soy-based formulas, will likely reveal more to scientists in years to come. In the meantime, doctors typically advise parents of hypothyroid infants not to give their babies soy-based formulas. But all parents should seriously consider whether they want to give their infants soy formulas until manufacturers have thoroughly and adequately addressed concerns about the isoflavone component of these products.

Dr. Fitzpatrick believes that people with hypothyroidism should seriously consider avoiding soy products, and predicts the current promotion of soy as a health food will result in an increase in thyroid disorders.

It's unfortunate that awareness of this serious concern isn't greater, and that authorities haven't taken the necessary steps to study and minimize this obvious health concern. The soy industry in the U.S. also does not appear to be actively recognizing the clear threat that soy products can represent to the thyroid.

RESEARCH PRIORITIES—BACTERIAL AND VIRAL CAUSES, ENVIRONMENTAL CONCERNS, TOXIC EXPOSURES

The study of bacteria as a cause of chronic diseases is just starting to gain momentum, but these sorts of investigations certainly should include thyroid disease. Just as scientists now know that ulcers and certain forms of heart disease can result from bacterial exposure, there is growing evidence that some autoimmune diseases have a bacterial component. Imagine if some forms of thyroid disease could be cured with an antibiotic or even prevented by a vaccine. It would be a revolutionary finding for many millions of people. This research needs to be a top priority.

At the same time, throughout this book, we've discussed the anecdotal link between the Epstein-Barr/mononucleosis virus and the development of autoimmune hypothyroidism. While research has yet to document a clear and obvious link between the Epstein-Barr virus and thyroid problems, this is an area that deserves extensive study. In addition, the search for other viral causes and links, and possible antiviral agents or vaccines, should also be a research priority.

Finally, the issue of toxic chemicals and their ability to negatively affect thyroid and endocrine function is also an area that needs far more in-depth study and research. While I touched upon some of the chemical exposure "risk factors" in chapter 2, many people don't realize how pervasive these concerns are and how many of us probably suffer from thyroid problems that stem from toxic environmental exposures.

Perchlorate, for example, a chemical used in rocket fuel and fireworks production, is a far greater concern than officials typically reveal. Perchlorate was manufactured near Henderson, Nevada. Specifically, there is concern that there is perchlorate contaminated groundwater feeding the Las Vegas Wash, Lake Mead, and into the Colorado River system. There is now evidence that perchlorate has reached the Central Arizona Project canal, which carries water from the California line to Phoenix and Tucson. Recently, perchlorate-contaminated drinking water has been discovered in dozens of communities around the country, not just in the southwest, raising the concern even further. In some areas where perchlorate concentrations are high, the rates of congenital hypothyroidism are substantially higher than normal, indicating that perchlorate-contaminated water may even be having an effect *in utero*.

The understanding of how long-term exposure to various chemicals affects the thyroid is really just beginning. Scientists are just now documenting the ability of certain chemicals to affect our endocrine glands and the thyroid in particular. But there's definitely evidence that exposure to certain chemicals increases the risk of developing thyroid disease.

Endocrine disruptors are man-made chemicals that mimic thyroid, estrogen, testosterone, and other hormones and, thus, affect the endocrine system, including the thyroid gland and its function. They also cause birth defects, cancer, infertility, and other serious health problems. The Endocrine Disruptor Screening and Testing Advisory Committee (EDSTAC) of the U.S. Environmental Protection Agency says that about *15,0000 different chemicals* that are included in common products like pesticides, cosmetics, and plastics should be analyzed to see if they act as endocrine disrupters. Internationally known health researcher and author Dr. Theodora Colborn, author of the book *Our Stolen Future*, believes that exposure to even low doses of endocrine disruptors can be harmful to our health. Coburn says:

> They're in lipstick, in the cosmetics you put on, in the solvents you clean house with, in fire retardants. These things are everywhere, and we know nothing about them.

Some researchers are now speculating that consistent postwar exposure to many synthetic chemicals that are foreign to our bodies may be causing a variety of toxic health affects, including thyroid problems, reproductive difficulties, and other increasingly common diseases and cancers.

Pesticides and dioxins are known to affect the thyroid. Frighteningly, even commercial nonorganic baby foods are known to contain what some deem unacceptable levels of dioxins. Another problem is Methyl Tertiary Butyl Ether, known as MTBE. MTBE is added to gasoline in high concentrations to increase octane levels, enhance combustion and improve air quality. The Environmental Protection Agency classifies MTBE, which can contaminate water supplies, as a possible human carcinogen because laboratory animals exposed to it have developed thyroid tumors, among other problems.

Scientists are still in the process of researching and documenting the specific relationships between chemical exposure and various illnesses, as well as the levels of exposure and time involved in order for exposures to be considered dangerous. But these are not just issues for scientists and environmental activists. We all need to make these concerns a priority. Environmental exposure may be at the root of our thyroid problems and the environment may pose an even greater danger to the thyroid and endocrine function of our children as well.

Find out what sorts of chemicals are being released into your neighborhood, and take a look at what types of health effects they have. You can find out more at the Chemical Scorecard Web site, *http://www.scorecard.org*.

THE RISE OF PATIENTS

Until now, hypothyroidism has never been a disease that garnered much attention from the media or even from patients. Until recently, thyroid patients who did not feel well on the standard treatment suffered in silence, unaware that they were not the only ones who were still plagued by a list of symptoms and health problems despite normal TSH values and treatment with levothyroxine. Now, the rise of the Internet, online support groups, bulletin boards, email, and newsletters have allowed for the dissemination of information not developed or funded by pharmaceutical companies and their related doctor and patient groups. And this revolution in information is reaching out beyond the Internet, by a variety of means—such as in books like this, newsletters, and other informational materials—that help patients learn more about their condition, connect with others, and stay up-to-date on the latest news and information.

The result is that a hypothyroid person today may actually know *more* than his or her doctor about hypothyroidism and the treatment options, better understand proper management of TSH levels, and have a much greater knowledge of the various tests beyond the TSH level to diagnose and evaluate thyroid function.

The power that knowledge and information offer to us as patients is a power we must exercise, if anything is to change. We must continue to speak out, make others aware, insist on representation from our legislators and patient groups, fight against overcharging by drug manufacturers, and keep asking for the research and answers we deserve.

Patients need to keep speaking up. Write the Thyroid Foundation of America, keep asking your doctor questions, write your legislators and the National Institutes of Health and ask them why more research isn't being conducted on thyroid disease, write your HMO, your local newspapers, Oprah, anyone who can help get the word out.

Patients need to expect more, demand more, and insist on

proper treatment and further research. It's the only way that many of us, and future generations, will ever move beyond the limitations imposed on our health and our lives by hypothyroidism and get on to the most important business of living well.

I encourage you to write me anytime with questions, thoughts, ideas, comments about the book, or if you want to share your personal story or experiences with hypothyroidism. You can reach me by email at mshomon@thyroid-info.com, or regular mail, at P.O. Box 0385, Palm Harbor, FL 34682.

Our education about thyroid disease doesn't stop here. This book is just one early effort in what should be an ongoing search for answers, information, and new developments to help diagnose, treat, and even potentially cure hypothyroidism. Every day, I review medical journals, news sources, Web sites, and conventional and alternative health resources, looking for information that can be of help to people with thyroid disease. Each month brings new developments in the search for conventional and alternative solutions for thyroid patients, information that can help you continue your efforts to live well with thyroid disease. I feature links to the best of this new information on the Web, and summarize important information at my Web site, www.thyroid-info.com.

I also publish key information and news in my monthly newsletter, *Sticking Out Our Necks*. Each issue of *Sticking Out Our Necks* features the kind of advice you've found in this book—knowledge you won't find assembled in one place anywhere else. You'll read about the newest thyroid-related ideas in complementary and alternative medicine. You'll discover exciting new ideas for better diagnosis, treatment, symptom relief, overall health, and empowerment for people with thyroid problems. You'll find more tips on the latest information that will help you effectively lose weight, stop hair loss, improve fertility, minimize allergies, and much more. Reader questions, stories, and letters will make you feel less alone in your journey on the road to living well with thyroid disease.

To order your subscription to *Sticking Out Our Necks*, write P.O. Box 0385, Palm Harbor, FL 34682, or call toll-free at 1-888-810-9471 (order processing only). Or visit www.thyroid-info.com for more information.

APPENDIX

RESOURCES

Personally, I felt an essential mission of this book was to assemble a list of useful resources to help you find the information and support you need regarding your hypothyroidism, thyroid disease, and health.

Resources sections, are, by their very nature, subject to change. You may, therefore, run into a phone number, or Web address that has changed since publication. If you come across out-of-date information and would like the updated information, please visit my Web site—http://www.thyroid-info.com. At the site, you'll find current listings for organizations and their contact information, current Web site addresses, links to online sources where you can get more information about any books that are mentioned, and other helpful resources.

If you just have email access, you can get an updated resources listing by emailing me at mshomon@thyroid-info.com, or if you don't have Web or email access at home, work, or library, please feel free to write to me at: Mary Shomon, P.O. Box 0385, Palm Harbor, FL 34682

STICKING OUT OUR NECKS—THE THYROID PATIENT NEWSLETTER

Sticking Out Our Necks is my newsletter, designed to keep thyroid patients up-to-date on important thyroid-related and health news— both conventional and alternative—that affects your ability to live well. I scour the health wires, medical journals, and alternative medicine sources—in the U.S. and around the world—looking for information that promises better diagnosis, treatment, and symptom relief for people with thyroid problems. Special articles look at the latest information on weight loss with hypothyroidism or up-to-the-minute news on the thyroid drugs and their manufacturers, your inspiring letters and testimonials about the solutions you are finding that help you live well, in-depth looks at linkages between thyroid and allergies, thyroid and fertility, and much more. A unique feature of *Sticking Out Our Necks* is the regular reporting on new developments in complementary and alternative medicine that have promise in dealing with all facets of thyroid disease, as well as treatment for unresolved thyroid symptoms. Finally, unlike other patient-oriented newsletters, *Sticking Out Our Necks* has no affiliations with any pharmaceutical companies or patient groups. This leaves me free to be honest and up front, telling it like it is about thyroid drugs and treatments and pharmaceutical company politics that have an impact on *your* quality of life. Each issue features eight pages packed full of news and information similar to what you've found in this book, information that helps you live well.

Free news highlights from *Sticking Out Our Necks* are available via email and online. Visit my book and newsletter Web site, http://www.thyroid-info.com, for more information.

NORTH AMERICAN THYROID-RELATED ORGANIZATIONS

Thyroid Foundation of America
Ruth Sleeper Hall RSL 350, 40 Parkman Street, Boston, MA 02114-2698
Phone: 1-800-832-8321, 617-726-8500 Fax: 617-726-4136
Email: tfa@clark.net
Web sites: http://www.tfaweb.org/pub/tfa, http://www.tsh.org

This is the main U.S. organization involved in thyroid education and outreach. Primarily run by doctors and medical interests, and funded in part by pharmaceutical companies, this organization stays fairly close to the official party line, but does offer decent conventional introductory information on thyroid disease and hypothyroidism.

MAGIC Foundation
1327 N. Harlem Avenue, Oak Park, IL 60302
Phone: 708-383-0808 Fax: 708-383-0899
Email: kacherkes@aol.com
Web sites: http://www.magicfoundation.org/clinhypo.html
http://members.tripod.com/~TDmagicmom/main.html
For information on infants and children with hypothyroidism, I recommend the MAGIC Foundation (Major Aspects of Growth In Children) for Children's Growth and Related Adult Disorders. Kelly Cherkes, their Thyroid Division Director, provided much of the information featured in the book on hypothyroidism in infants and children. This Chicago-based organization was established in 1989 and is a national nonprofit 501(c)(3) providing support and education regarding growth disorders in children and related adult disorders, including adult growth hormone disorder. MAGIC's membership has grown from twenty to more than 6,000. The MAGIC network covers 100 types of growth disorders, ten specific divisions—including thyroid disease—and educational/supportive services worldwide. MAGIC offers educational brochures, national networking for parents, an annual national convention, and a quarterly newsletter, *The MAGIC Touch,* which covers medical updates, personal stories and organization-related information for all divisions.

American Foundation for Thyroid Patients
P.O. Box 820195, Houston, TX 77282
Email: thyroid@flash.net
Web site: http://www.thyroidfoundation.org/
A patient founded this thyroid organization, which offers a newsletter and other support.

Thyroid Society for Education and Research
7515 South Main Street, Suite 545, Houston, TX 77030
Phone: 1-800-THYROID Fax: 713-799-9919
Email: help@the-thyroid-society.org
Web site: http://www.the-thyroid-society.org
This small organization has a conventional focus and is run by a doctor. They offer doctor referrals via mail and a quarterly newsletter for supporters and donors.

National Graves' Disease Foundation
2 Tsitsi Court, Brevard, NC 28712
Phone: 704-877-5251 Fax: 704-877-5251
Email: ngdf@citcom.net
Web site: http://www.ngdf.org
    This group has a fairly conventional focus. Key activities include an educational conference for patients.

Thyroid Cancer Survivor's Organization and Conference
ThyCa, P.O. Box 1545, New York, NY 10159-1545
Phone: 877-588-7904 (toll-free) Fax: 503-905-9725
Email: thyca@thyca.org
Web site: http://www.thyca.org
    Known as ThyCa this patient-founded and focused organization provides information and support to survivors of thyroid cancer and their families. They hold an annual conference and sponsor a popular patient support listserv. A very patient-oriented, top-quality group.

Thyroid Foundation of Canada/La Fondation
Canadienne de la Thyroide
96 Mack Street, Kingston, Ontario K7L 1N9 Canada
Phone: 613-544-8364 Fax: 613-544-9731
Email: thyroid@limestone.kosone.com
Web site: http://home.ican.net/~thyroid/Canada.html
    Canada's top thyroid education-related organization for patients.

THYROID ORGANIZATIONS OUTSIDE
NORTH AMERICA

Diana Holmes
Plot B, Sunnybank, Lapley South Staffordshire, UK ST19 9QH
Phone: 01785 841 449
E-mail: dianaholmes@barclays.net
    In her book *Tears Behind Closed Doors,* published in England, Diana Holmes tells her compelling account of years of misdiagnosis. Doctors finally discovered her hypothyroidism, despite normal TSH levels. Diana now provides support to her fellow U.K. thyroid sufferers.

British Thyroid Foundation
P.O. Box 97, Clifford Wetherby, West Yorks LS23 6XD United Kingdom

Thyroid Eye Disease Association
34 Fore Street, Chudleigh Devon TQ13 0HX United Kingdom
Phone: 44 1626 852980 Fax: 44 1626 852980
Web site: http://home.ican.net/~thyroid/International/TED.html

Thyroid Australia
PP Box 2575, Fitzroy Delivery Centre Melbourne, VIC 3065, Australia
Phone: 61 3 9561 3483 Fax: 61 3 9561 4798
E-mail: aalunste@bigpond.net.au

Australian Thyroid Foundation
Australia's P.O. Box 186, Westmead NSW 2145 Australia
Phone: 02-9890 6962 Fax: 02-9755 7073
Email: snewlands@bigpond.com

Thyreoidea Landsforeningen
c/o Lis Larsen Abakkevej 55, st. tv, 2720 Vanlose Denmark
Email: Lis_Larsen@net.dialog.dk

Schilddrusen Liga Deutschland e.V.
Postfach 800 740 65907 Frankfurt Germany
Phone: 49 69 31 40 53 76 Fax: 49 69 31 40 53 16
Web site: http://www.thyrolink.com/sd-liga

Associazione Italiana Basedowiani e Tiroidei
c/o Centro Minerva 7 Via Mazzini 43100 Parma Italy
Phone: 39 521-207771 Fax: 39 521-207771

Schildklierstichting Nederland
Postbus 138, 1620 AC Hoorn, Holland

Vastsvenska Patientforeningen for Skoldkortelsjoka
Mejerivalen 8, 439 36 Onsala, Sweden
Phone: 46 30 06 39 12 Fax: 46 30 06 39 12

SUPPORT GROUPS

The Thyroid Foundation of America and the British Thyroid Foundation keep track of various patient interest groups and will assist you if you wish to start your own thyroid support group.

The Thyroid Cancer Survivor's Organization has local area support groups. See their Web site, http://www.thyca.org, for more information.

Thyroid Top Docs Directory (see http://www.thyroid-info.com) features support group information on state-by-state and international page listings.

The Magic Foundation organizes support groups for parents of children with thyroid problems. Contact them for more information.

Internet-based Thyroid Support Groups

There are several key online support areas for thyroid disease, the Usenet newsgroup alt.support.thyroid, the bulletin boards at my About.com Web site, http://www.delphi.com/ab-thyroid, and AOL's various boards and chats on thyroid disease, as well as a number of other key chat and boards areas at other sites.

Because information changes so frequently for the various boards and chats, for the latest list of Web-based support information, please visit my Web site at http://www.thyroid-info.com

FINDING AND VERIFYING DOCTORS AND THEIR CREDENTIALS

Thyroid Top Docs Directory
Web site: http://www.thyroid-info.com
A free state-by-state and international listing of top doctors for thyroid disease. Doctors are recommended by other thyroid patients and listings often feature detailed information on why the particular doctor was recommended. There are some truly excellent doctors on this list, and several of the practitioners featured in this book were found via the *Top Docs Directory*.

Thyroid Foundation of America (TFA)
TFA (see the previous section "North American Thyroid-Related Organizations") offers referrals to doctors who specialize in thyroid disease. There are some good doctors being referred by TFA, but keep in mind, most referrals will be to highly conventional doctors.

American Association of Clinical Endocrinologists
1000 Riverside Ave.; Suite 205, Jacksonville, FL 32204
Phone: 904-353-7878, Fax: 904-353-8185
Web site: http://www.aace.com
The American Association of Clinical Endocrinologists (AACE) is a profes-

sional medical organization devoted to clinical endocrinology. At their Web site they sponsor an online "Specialist Search Page," at http://www.aace.com/directory, which allows you to identify AACE members by geographic location, including international options. A unique feature is the ability to select by subspecialty. Again, as a mainstream organization of endocrinologists, expect mainly conventional approaches from these referrals.

Thyroid Foundation of Canada/La Fondation
Canadienne de la Thyroïde
(see the previous section "North American Thyroid-Related Organizations") The Thyroid Foundation of Canada offers referrals for doctors in Canada. Again, you're likely to find conventional doctors via this organization.

MAGIC (Major Aspects of Growth In Children)
Foundation for Children's Growth
(see the previous section "North American Thyroid-Related Organizations") MAGIC provides referrals to top pediatric endocrinologists. MAGIC relies on parents' recommendations in part, so you're likely to get decent referrals to good pediatric thyroid specialists.

Broda Barnes Research Foundation
P.O. Box 98, Trumbull, CT 06611
Phone: 203-261-2101 Fax: 203-261-3017
Email: info@BrodaBarnes.org
Web site: http://www.brodabarnes.org
   This organization was founded to advance the theories and approaches begun by Dr. Broda Barnes during his career. If you're interested in finding a doctor who applies the Barnes Basal Metabolism Approach to diagnosing thyroid disease, you might want to contact this group. Some people have reported finding excellent, openminded doctors they love through this organization. For a $10.00 fee, they'll send you a package of informational articles and materials, and information on doctors who practice using their approaches, and I know there are some good doctors on their lists. But I recommend that you ask any doctors referred to you by this organization right up front if they have a required battery of expensive tests that they insist on before treatment. If so, ask about the tests, how much they cost, and what the initial consultation fee is for a new patient. Some people have complained that the doctors they were referred to from this organization seemed more interested in getting the patients in for $300-$400 initial consultations, plus $500 or more in lab fees for all kinds of tests no one has ever heard of, supposedly sending blood, urine, saliva, and hair samples all over the world at high cost. So definitely ask questions before you even schedule your first appointment.

Moving on to the more general services, not specific to the thyroid world, there are a number of referral and verification sources to investigate.

American Osteopathic Association
142 East Ontario Street, Chicago, IL 60611
Phone: 800-621-1773, Fax: 312-202-8200
Email: www@aoa.nat.org
Web site: http://www.am-osteo-assn.org
   The American Osteopathic Association has state referral lists for osteopaths in all 50 states.

American Board of Medical Specialties "Certified Doctor" Service
Phone: 800-776-2378
Web site: http://www.certifieddoctor.org
   This is an online service that allows you to browse for conventional doctors by specialty and locale and get certification info on specific docs.

American Medical Association (AMA) "Physician Select"
Web site: http://www.ama-assn.org/aps/amahg.htm
   The AMA's Physician Select program allows you to browse their database for AMA member doctors, almost always conventional doctors. It lists medical school and year graduated, residency training, primary practice, secondary practice, major professional activity, and board certification for all doctors who are licensed physicians.

American Holistic Health Association
P.O. Box 17400, Anaheim, CA 92817-7400
Phone: (714) 779-6152
Email: ahha@healthy.net
Web site: http://www.ahha.org/
Searchable database of practitioners: http://www.healthy.net/aspAssociations/assocsearch.asp?table=American+Holistic+Health+Association
   The American Holistic Health Association offers an online referral to its members, who are holistic doctors.

American Holistic Medical Association
6728 Old McLean Village Drive, McLean, VA 22101
Phone: 703-556-9728 Fax: 703-556-8729
Patient Information number: 1-703-556-9728.
Email: HolistMed@aol.com
Web site: http://www.ahmaholistic.com
   The American Holistic Medical Association publishes a Referral Directory of member M.D.s and D.O.s.

Dr. Andrew Weil's Practitioner Database

http://cgi.pathfinder.com/drweil/practitioner/search/1,2020,,00.html

I *know* this online service from alternative medicine guru Andrew Weil is a good database, because my personal physician, who is an M.D. and acupuncturist, is in there, as are her partners in practice, osteopaths who also practice acupuncture and physiatry. Great resource for searching for doctors by state, zip code, or area code in a variety of complementary approaches.

1-800-DOCTORS and Similar Services

Many areas have telephone-based doctor referral services. For example, 1-800-DOCTORS allows you to call up and obtain information on doctors in your area. You can also find out which conventional doctors in their system match up to your healthcare program. 1-800-DOCTORS operates in a number of major markets, including Chicago; Washington, DC; Dallas/Fort Worth; Denver; Houston; Milwaukee; and Philadelphia; and many cities have similar services. Check your yellow pages.

Hospital Referrals

If a hospital in your area has a referral service, this can be a decent source of information and referrals to doctors. If the hospital's reputation is good, the doctors typically are going to be of a better caliber. Some of the more sophisticated hospital referral services will offer educational and practice style information about doctors in their databases.

U.S. News and World Report "Best Graduate Schools"/Medical School Evaluation

Phone: 1-800-836-6397

Web site: http://www.usnews.com/usnews/edu/beyond/gradrank/med/gdmedt1.htm

You can evaluate whether or not your doctor went to a good medical school by checking the med school rankings provided by *U.S. News and World Report*. The information is available on the Web and you can also order their *Best Graduate Schools*, a $5.95 directory, at the Web site or by calling their 800 number.

Doctor Ratings

Find out if any of your local magazines rate doctors. *Washingtonian* magazine, for example, periodically asks doctors to pick those other Washington, DC/Maryland/Virginia area doctors they'd most recommend in particular specialties and publishes the results. It's always a comfort to me to see a doctor I've been referred to appear on this list, although it doesn't always guarantee I'll *like* that doctor!

Best Doctors

Phone: 1-888-DOCTORS

Web site: http://www.bestdoctors.com

Best Doctors has a Family Doc-Finder at their Web site where, for a small fee, you can find recommended primary care physicians in your area. You'll find only conventional doctors via this service. Best Doctors also conducts specialized physician searches for rare, catastrophic, or serious illnesses. The specialized search costs $1,500, only called for in the direst situations, but it's worth knowing about if you find yourself seriously in need of a specialist or expert.

Questionable Doctors Listing
Web site: http://www.citizen.org/hrg/MAJORPUBLICATIONS/qdform.htm
Check on whether your doctor has been listed in the "16,638 Questionable Doctors," report, which was produced by the consumer advocacy group Public Citizen. The book lists 16,638 doctors who were disciplined by state medical boards or federal agencies. Among these doctors were those accused of sexual abuse, substandard care, incompetence or negligence, criminal conviction, misprescribing drugs, and substance abuse. Interestingly, up to 69 percent of these doctors disciplined are still practicing medicine. You can order the report for your state or region for $20 by phone or at the Web site.

Medical Board Charges or Actions
You can also find out if disciplinary action has even been taken with your doctor or if charges are pending against him or her, by calling your state Medical Board. A good list of all medical boards is found at http://www.fsmb.org/members.htm, and you can also search at the Association of State Medical Board Executive Directors, "DocFinder," service, http://www.docboard.org/.

COMPANIES MANUFACTURING THYROID HORMONE REPLACEMENT FOR SALE IN THE U.S.

Levoxyl and Cytomel
Jones Pharma
1945 Craig Road St. Louis, MO 63146
Phone: 800-525-8466 Fax: 314-469-5749
Information: Contact Customer Service at 800-525-8466
Email: jmedpharma@mindspring.com
Web site: http://www.jmedpharma.com
Levoxyl is a levothyroxine product. Cytomel is liothyronine, the synthetic form of triiodothyronine (T3). Their public information staff and pharmacists are friendly and extremely helpful, and this company is always willing to provide information and assistance to patients.

Armour Thyroid, Thyrolar, Levothroid

Forest Pharmaceuticals
Professional Affairs Department
13600 Shoreline Drive, St Louis, MO 63045
Phone: 800-678-1605, x 7037 Fax: 314-493-7457
Email: dwesche@forestpharm.com
Web site: http://www.forestpharm.com/

Armour Thyroid is a natural thyroid hormone replacement product. Thyrolar is the brand name for liotrix, synthetic T4/T3 levothyroxine/liothyronine combination drug. Levothroid is a levothyroxine drug. Forest has consistently been very proactive in making sure that their customers have access to information and have been extremely helpful and supportive to patients. (Note: Currently, Armour Thyroid and Thyrolar are not readily available outside the U.S. If you are interested in these products in Canada or other countries, start by contacting the Broda Barnes Foundation.)

Westhroid/Naturethroid

Western Research Laboratories
12209 North 32nd Street, Phoenix, Arizona 85032
Phone: 602-482-9370 Fax: 602-482-8889

Westhroid is a cornstarch-bound, natural thyroid hormone product, made from desiccated pig thyroid gland. Naturethroid is also made from desiccated pig thyroid gland, but as it is bound with microcrystalline cellulose, it is hypoallergenic. Both products are available from Western Research Laboratories, which was part of Jones Pharma and is now an independent company. Westhroid and Naturethroid are sold directly to doctors and pharmacies in the U.S. and Canada. Patients can get a list of doctors in their areas who use these products by contacting the company directly. The folks at Western are very friendly and interested in making sure that patients and doctors feel free to call anytime with questions and requests for more information.

Synthroid

Knoll Pharmaceutical Medical Information Department
3000 Continental Drive, North Mount Olive, NJ 07828
Phone: 1-800-526-0221
Web site: http://www.synthroid.com

Knoll's hotline is not the most helpful. The company that is so willing to sell you Synthroid has created one of those voice mail systems that makes it almost impossible to get any information.

Note Regarding Synthroid Lawsuit/Litigation: At the time of publication, a recorded message regarding the Synthroid Lawsuit was available at 1-800-254-3079. The plaintiff's attorney support line for Synthroid litigation, which is the only way to attempt to speak with a live person regarding the lawsuit, was 1-800-853-4853. Updated numbers and information on the lawsuit are available at my Web site and will also be published in my news report as any new number or information becomes available.

THYROID-SPECIFIC WEB SITES

Thyroid Information Central—http://www.thyroid-info.com
Home page for this book, and for my monthly news report, *Sticking Out Our Necks*. You'll find thyroid news and information, personal thyroid stories, and more. The site has hundreds of comprehensive, up-to-date links to the Web's best resources on hypothyroidism, thyroid disease, and health information.

Thyroid Disease at About.com—http://thyroid.about.com
This is my Thyroid Disease Web site at About.com (formerly the Mining Company), where you'll find dozens of feature articles related to all facets of thyroid disease, in-depth annotated links to hundreds of the Web's best thyroid disease sites, and my popular thyroid bulletin boards and twenty-four-hour-a-day chatroom, where you can exchange information and support with other people with thyroid disease.

Endocrineweb—http://www.endocrineweb.com
A large site developed by doctors with more in-depth information on thyroid disease. Conventional focus but good depth of information, especially on surgery.

Thyroid Disease Manager—http://www.thyroidmanager.org
Full-length book offering detailed, highly conventional thyroid information with a medical tone and focus, primarily for doctors.

Thyroid Foundation of America (TFA)—http://www.tsh.org and http://www.clark.net/pub/tfa
Decent selection of basic conventional information on thyroid disease.

Thyroid Foundation of Canada—http://home.ican.net/~thyroid/ Canada.html
Good collection of conventional information, article reprints, and patient publications on thyroid disease.

THYROID-RELATED BOOKS

There are a number of conventional thyroid books written by doctors, and frankly I'm not even going to recommend them here at all. I find them sometimes condescending, too similar to each other, and consistent in presenting a narrow, conventional, doctor-oriented— instead of patient-oriented—view. These are the books that I do recommend that can be of help in covering certain aspects of thyroid disease or hypothyroidism:

The Thyroid Solution: A Mind-Body Program for Beating Depression and Regaining Your Emotional and Physical Health
Ridha Arem, M.D.

Unlike the other currently available patient-directed books on thyroid disease, Dr. Arem, an endocrinologist, talks honestly and openly about symptoms such as brain fog, depression, loss of libido, weight gain, anxiety, and many others. Arem's strongest suit is in his research and analysis of the relationship of thyroid disease to brain chemistry, and resulting depression, anxiety disorders, mood disorders, and other mental and emotional effects of hypothyroidism.

The Thyroid Sourcebook
M. Sara Rosenthal

The third edition of this book fills an important niche in patients' general thyroid information needs. It offers a good cross-section of information on thyroid disease, including cancer, nodules, goiters, autoimmune disease, hyperthyroidism and hypothyroidism, among others. The book's strength is in its conventional details. Don't expect any discussion of alternative or unconventional topics, however.

Tears Behind Closed Doors
Diana Holmes

This book, published in England in 1998, is one woman's account that would sound very familiar to many people reading this book. Diana was misdiagnosed six different times with everything from celiac disease to myasthenia gravis and, ultimately, was found to have hypothyroidism, despite TSH levels in the "normal range." Diana tells her own moving and empowering account in the hope that her story will help others.

Hypothyroidism: The Unsuspected Illness
Broda Otto Barnes, M.D.

This book, published back in 1982, was written by the now-deceased Dr. Broda Barnes. It is considered the bible for alternative thyroid information and

---

use of basal body temperature in diagnosis. The book is still in print but not likely to be stocked in bookstores. It is, however, available by special order, or at the Web's online bookstores. The book contains a fair amount of out-of-date information, but it is the first to truly acknowledge the wide-ranging impact the thyroid has on nearly every facet of health. Also, it doesn't talk down to patients or dismiss various health concerns.

Solved: The Riddle of Illness
Stephen Langer, M.D., James F. Scheer

Langer, a follower of Broda Barnes' theories, has written what he calls the followup to Barnes' book. It looks at some nutritional and vitamin approaches for hypothyroidism. It still feels like a doctor telling the patient what to do and doesn't address in any depth the problems of getting a diagnosis, dealing with doctors, and dealing with depression. The book is at its best discussing supplements and nutritional approaches that might help hypothyroidism. This book is out of print but may still be available in used bookstores.

DOCTORS AND PRACTITIONERS WHO CONTRIBUTED TO THIS BOOK

Dr. Zafirah Ahmed, Ph.D., N.D.
Private office: Dr. Ahmed's Center for Natural Healing
500 W. Broadway #113, Tempe, AZ 85282
Phone: 602-267-7349 Fax: 602-225-5144
Clinic: International Health Clinic
2855 E. Brown Rd. #17, Mesa AZ 85213
Phone: 602-218-7110 Fax: 602-218-7106
Email: drahmed@primenet.com, hakimaz@ivillage.com

Kenneth Blanchard, M.D.
2000 Washington Street, Suite 565, Newton Lower Falls, MA 02462
Phone: 617-527-1810

Dana Godbout Laake, M.S., R.D.H., L.N.
11140 Rockville Pike, Suite 600, Rockville, MD 20852
Phone: 301-998-6575 Fax: 301-984-6559
Email: danalaake@erols.com

Kate Lemmerman, M.D.
Kaplan Clinic
5275 Lee Highway, Suite 200, Arlington, VA 22207

Phone: 703-532-4892
Web site: http://www.kaplanclinic.com

Sandra Levy, M.S., C.M.T.
Alexandria Myotherapy
333 North Fairfax St., Suite 303, Alexandria, VA 22314
Phone: 703-548-2270
Web site: http://www.alexmyo.com

John C. Lowe, M.A., D.C., A.A.P.M.
Pain Management Specialist, Fibromyalgia and Hypothyroidism Researcher
P.O. Box 396, Tulsa, OK 74101-0396
Phone: 918-582-7733
Email: jlowe55555@aol.com
Web site: http://www.drlowe.com
    (While Dr. Lowe focuses his efforts on research and education, his partner
and wife, Dr. Gina Honeyman-Lowe, accepts patients for treatment under the
protocols he developed. She can be reached at the same address and phone
number, Email: ghoneyman@aol.com)

Susan Osborne, D.O.
110 North Locust Street, Floyd, VA 24091
Phone: 540-745-6034
Email: family_stephens@hotmail.com

Patricia Rackowski
    Host of "Menopause: Let's Talk About It" workshops on self-help for
menopause, choices in hormone replacement therapy, traditional herbs for
menopause, and sexual desire in menopause.
Email: prackowski@erols.com
Web site: http://www.menopause-consultant.com

Cynthia White
Aerobic Instructor/Personal Trainer
Denton, Texas
Phone: 940-440-9130

COMPLEMENTARY AND ALTERNATIVE THERAPIES FOR HYPOTHYROIDISM

Acupuncture

American Association of Oriental Medicine
433 Front St., Catasauqua, PA 18032
Phone: 610-266-1433 Fax: 610-264-2768

Email: AAOM1@aol.com
Web site: http://www.aaom.org

AAOM provides referrals to practitioners who are state-licensed or certified by various respected certifying organizations. They also have an online state-by-state referral search for TCM and acupuncture practitioners at http://www.aaom.org/referral.html.

**National Certification Commission for
Acupuncture and Oriental Medicine**
Department 0595, Washington, DC 20073-0595
Phone: 202-232-1404

NCCAOM awards the title Dipl.Ac. to acupuncture practitioners who pass its certification requirements. You can get a list of Diplomates of Acupuncture in your state for $3.

American Academy of Medical Acupuncture
Phone: 800-521-2262

The AAMA, which provides referrals, requires that its members—who are all physicians—undergo at least 220 hours of continuing medical education in acupuncture.

Accreditation Commission for Acupuncture and Oriental Medicine
Phone: 301-608-9680

This organization can verify which American schools of acupuncture and Oriental medicine have reliable reputations.

Acupuncture.com
Web site: http://www.acupuncture.com/Referrals/ref2.htm

Acupuncture.com offers a list of licensed acupuncturists by state.

Ayurveda

The Maharishi Ayurveda Medical Center
Phone: 800-248-9050, 800-255-8332 Fax: 719-260-7400

Provides information on ayurveda as well as referrals to ayurvedic practitioners.

Herbal Medicine

It doesn't hurt to start with a good overview of herbal medicine. I highly recommend *Herbal Defense,* by Robyn Landis, with Karta Purkh Singh Khalsa, published in 1997. Robyn also has a Web site located at http://www.bodyfueling.com/ with a variety of herbal information.

Herb Research Foundation
1007 Pearl Street, Suite 200, Boulder, CO 80302
Phone: 800-748-2617 Herbal Hotline: 303-449-2265
Web site: http://www.herbs.org
    More information on herbal support, specifically for thyroid function, is available in a detailed packet, $7 for nonmembers. Individual memberships are also available for $35 a year and include a free information packet and a subscription to the foundation's magazine. To order a packet or find out more about membership, contact: Herb Research Foundation at 303-449-2265. They also have a specialized Herbal Hotline to answer specific questions, for a small fee, usually less than $10. You need a Visa/Mastercard to use this service.

Nutritional and Vitamin Therapy

Many people read up on the various vitamin therapies and treat themselves using vitamins and minerals. This is a very common form of self-care. If you choose to self-treat, I'd urge you to get a copy of two key books:

Prescription for Nutritional Healing
by James F. Balch, M.D. and Phyllis A. Balch
    I consider this book the ultimate reference source for information on various natural approaches to disease and health problems. Part One reviews nutrients, food supplements, and herbal supplements. Part Two reviews various disorders and recommended nutritional treatments. Part Three covers other remedies and therapies. Before you buy another vitamin or herb, get a copy of this book.

8 Weeks to Optimum Health
Andrew Weil, M.D.
    This book is by Andrew Weil, alternative medicine's current guru and spokesperson. Dr. Weil's book outlines an excellent eight-week, step-by-step guide to building up and nourishing the mind, body, and spirit, and restoring energy and resilience to the immune system. His recommendations range from adding various supplements to your diet to going on a "news fast" periodically. Dr. Weil's suggestions are practical, doable, and surprisingly effective.
    You can also see Dr. Weil's Web site, http://www.drweil.com, for an excellent Vitamin Advisor and database.

American Dietetic Association's Nationwide Nutrition Network
Phone: 800-366-1655
Web database: http://www.eatright.org/finddiet.html
    This organization offers referrals to registered dietitians and a searchable online database of registered dietitians.

Naturopathy

American Association of Naturopathic Physicians
2366 Eastlake Avenue East, Suite 322, Seattle, Washington 98102
Phone: 206-323-7610 Referral Line: 206-298-0125
Web site database: http://www.naturopathic.org/FindND.html
    This group offers a referral line, directory, and brochures that explain naturopathic medicine. I believe the fee for this directory is $5.

Manual Healing and Bodywork

National Certification Board for Therapeutic Massage and Bodywork
Phone: 703-524-9563 or 800-296-0664
    This organization provides names of bodywork therapists certified by the board.

American Massage Therapy Association
Phone: 708-864-0123
    This group offers only information on massage therapy and referrals to therapists who are members of AMTA.

Associated Bodywork & Massage Professionals
Phone: 303-674-8478 Referral Line: 800-458-2267
    This organization offers referrals to bodywork practitioners.

Osteopathic Manipulation

American Osteopathic Association
142 East Ontario Street, Chicago, IL 60611
Phone: 1-800-621-1773 Fax: 312-202-8200
Email: www@aoa.nat.org
Web site: http://www.am-osteo-assn.org
    The association has state referral lists for all 50 states and can provide additional information on osteopathic medicine.

Mind/Body Therapy

There are so many places you can look for mind-body practitioners, everything from psychotherapists to ministers to yogis to art therapists. Ask friends, check bulletin boards, or publications at your local health food store, even local alternative health or alternative newsweeklies, for ideas on how to find a good mind-body therapist.

For traditional mental health support, such as a psychologist, a counselor, or general support groups, contact:

National Mental Health Association
1021 Prince Street, Alexandria, VA 22314-2971
Phone: 800-969-NMHA
　　Provides referrals to state and regional mental health associations and resources.

National Mental Health Consumers Self-Help Clearinghouse
1211 Chestnut Street, Suite 1000, Philadelphia, PA 19107
Phone: 800-553-4539 Fax: 215-636-6310
Email: info@mhselfhelp.org
　　Offers articles and books on consumer-oriented and mental health issues; and a reference file on relevant groups, organizations, and agencies.

Canadian Mental Health Association
2160 Yonge Street, 3rd Floor, Toronto, Ontario M4S 2Z3
Phone: 416-484-7750 Fax: 416-484-4617
Email: cmhanat@interlog.com
Web site: http://www.icomm.ca/cmhacan/english/homeng.htm
　　Provides referrals to regional mental health associations and resources.

For other types of referrals, some of these organizations can help:

Center for Mind/Body Medicine
P.O. Box 1048, La Jolla, CA 92038
Phone: 619-794-2425 Fax: 619-794-2440
　　Developed under the guidance of Deepak Chopra, M.D., offers both residential and outpatient programs, as well as education and training programs in Ayurveda.

American Chronic Pain Association
P.O. Box 850, Rocklin, CA 95677
Phone: 916-632-0922
　　This group manages a list of over 500 support groups internationally and publishes workbooks and a newsletter.

Center for Attitudinal Healing
33 Buchanan, Sausalito, CA 94965

Phone: 415-331-6161

Support groups throughout the nation for people with chronic or serious illness.

Wellness Community
2716 Ocean Park Blvd., Suite 1040, Santa Monica, CA 90405
Phone: 310-314-2555

Chapters throughout the nation offer support groups for people with chronic or serious illness.

Phylameara Désy—Healing Expert
Web sites: http//www.spiralvisions.com
　　　　　http//www.healing.about.com

Excellent resource for information or all facts of mind-body healing and wellness.

Yoga

Yoga in Daily Life Center/US
1310 Mount Vernon Avenue, Alexandria, VA 22301
Phone: 703-299-8946 Fax: 703-299-9051
Email: yidl@erols.com, ashram@yoga-in-daily-life-usa.com
Web site: http://www.yoga-in-daily-life-usa.com

Offers yoga information and an extensive online book, video/audio, and supplies store. I highly recommend their "Yoga Nidra" relaxation tapes, and I practice yoga at home using their beginner video.

Yoga Journal
P.O. Box 12008, Berkeley, CA 94712-3008
Phone: 1-800-I-DO-YOGA
Web site: http://www.yogajournal.com/

This bimonthly magazine also publishes a directory of yoga teachers and organizations. Their Web site features an online directory of teachers.

YogaClass
Web site: http://yogaclass.com/

YogaClass offers free online yoga, relaxation, and breathing classes, presented in "RealPlayer" video/audio format.

YogaSite's Directory of Yoga Teachers
Web site: http://www.yogasite.com/teachers.html

This is a decent online directory of yoga teachers.

Homeopathy

National Center for Homeopathy
801 N Fairfax St. Suite 306, Alexandria, VA 22314-1757
Phone: 703-548-7790
Web site database: http://homeopathic.org/NCHSearch.htm.
This organization offers referrals, information on homeopathy, and an on-line referral database.

Aromatherapy

Herb Research Foundation
1007 Pearl Street, Suite 200, Boulder, CO 80302
Phone: 303-449-2265
More information on aromatherapy and herbal support for thyroid function is available from this group.

American Alliance of Aromatherapy
P.O. Box 309, Depoe Bay, OR 97341
Phone: 800-809-9850 Fax: 800-809-9808

National Association for Holistic Aromatherapy
P.O. Box 17622, Boulder, CO 80308
Phone: 800-566-6735

General Alternative Medicine Referral Sources

The following are multidisciplinary national referrals to alternative medicine practitioners.

American College for Advancement in Medicine
Web site: http://www.acam.org
This nonprofit medical society dedicated to educating physicians on the latest findings in complementary/alternative medicine has a searchable listing of ACAM physicians at their Web site.

HealthWorld Online's Professional Referral Network
Web site: http://www.healthy.net/clinic/refer/index.html
Offers referrals to practitioners of alternative and complementary medicine and integrative health care. Searchable referral databases for a variety of alternative modalities.

Dr. Andrew Weil's Practitioner Database
Web site: http://cgi.pathfinder.com/drweil/practitioner/search/index.html
   Excellent database of more than 10,000 alternative practitioners, searchable by state, zip code, or area code.

American Holistic Health Association
(see listing under "Finding and Verifying Doctors and Their Credentials")
   This organization offers referrals to a variety of certified holistic practitioners.

American Holistic Medical Association
(see listing under "Finding and Verifying Doctors and Their Credentials")
   This organization offers a Referral Directory for member M.D.s and D.O.s.

Well Mind Association
Phone: 301-774-6617
   Offers national referrals to over 700 alternative practitioners.

Alternative Medicine Yellow Pages: The Comprehensive Guide to the New World of Health
   This $12.95 book, edited by Melinda Bonk, and published by Future Medicine Publishing, is a national directory of over 17,000 practitioners of alternative medicine, sorted by specialties. Available at bookstores or online bookstores like Amazon.com or Barnes and Noble.
   While by no means a comprehensive list, some regions also have good referral services, including the following.

* DC, MD, VA: Alternative Medicine Referral Service. 301-220-HEAL. Free referrals to over 180 practitioners.
* AR, LA, OK, MO, and TX: Arklahoma Healing Arts Alliance, Inc, Phone: 501-785-2422. Free referrals to healthcare practitioners using alternative therapies.
* TX: WELLNET (Wholistic Referral Network), Phone: 800-520-WELL Fax: 972-479-0838. Free referrals to over 175 practitioners in Dallas/ Ft. Worth, Austin, and San Antonio areas.
* NJ: Holistic Health Association of the Princeton Area, Phone: 609-924-8580, Email: mandala@ix.netcom.com. Online referral list: http://www.holisticliving.org. Free referrals to over 5,000 healthcare practitioners in central New Jersey.
* AZ: International Holistic Center, Inc., Phone: 602-287-0605. Phone referrals, or you alternative practitioner directories for Phoenix and Prescott.
* CA (Los Angeles, Orange County): Natural Resource Directory, Phone: 310-305-8521, Email: aross@nrd.com Online directory: http://www.nrd.com. 150 practitioners in the Los Angeles/ Orange County, CA area.
* FL: New Radiance Metaphysical & Holistic Florida Directory, Phone: 813-

573-2661, Email: newradcorp@aol.com. They sell a statewide directory of alternative practitioners in Florida.

Alternative Medicine Content Web sites

Dr. Weil—http://www.drweil.com

A searchable alternative medicine database, interactive vitamin adviser, and alternative practitioner index make this one of the Web's premier alternative medicine resources.

Alternative Medicine Magazine— http://www.alternativemedicine.com

Full-text archive of this popular, well-done alternative medicine magazine. Features several excellent articles on alternative treatment for hypothyroidism.

HealthWorld Online—http://www.healthy.net/

Home page for extensive information on complementary and alternative medicine options in healthcare, including excellent data base of articles related to hypothyroidism.

Healthy Ideas—http://www.healthy.net/

Web site home page for *Prevention Magazine* uses the magazine's vitamin, nutrition, exercise, and self-care focus.

Gary Null's Natural Living—http://www.garynull.com

An excellent site that explores the nature and politics of medicine, health, nutrition, and the environment.

LOSING WEIGHT DESPITE HYPOTHYROIDISM

Recommended books and their Web sites include:

- *Becoming Vegetarian: The Complete Guide to Adopting a Healthy Vegetarian Diet*, by Vesanto Melina
- *The Zone: A Dietary Road Map to Lose Weight Permanently* and *Mastering the Zone: The Next Step in Achieving Superhealth and Permanent Fat Loss,* by Barry Sears
- *Fat Free, Flavor Full: Dr. Gabe Mirkin's Guide to Losing Weight and Living Longer*, by Dr. Gabe Mirkin
- *Dr. Bob Arnot's Revolutionary Weight Control Program*, by Dr. Bob Arnot
- *The G-Index Diet : The Missing Link That Makes Permanent Weight Loss Possible*, by Richard N. Podell, William Proctor
- *Dr. Tony Perrone's Body-Fat Breakthru*, by Dr. Tony Perrone

- *Weigh Less, Live Longer: Dr. Lou Aronne's 'Getting Healthy' Plan for Permanent Weight Control,* by Dr. Lou Aronne
- *Dr. Atkins' New Diet Revolution,* by Robert C. Atkins, M.D., 1-888-ATKINS-8
- *Sugar Busters! Cut Sugar to Trim Fat,* by H. Leighton Steward, Morrison C. Bethea, Sam S. Andrews

WEB SITES

- Vegetarianism—http://www.vegsource.com, http://vegetariancentral.org
- Weight Watchers—http://www.weightwatchers.com
- The Zone—http://www.enterthezone.com
- Dr. Gabe Mirkin—http://www.wdn.com/mirkin
- Atkins Diet—http://www.atkinscenter.com
- SugarBusters—http://www.sugarbusters.com

DEPRESSION AND HYPOTHYROIDISM

These organizations can provide more information, referrals, and support groups for depression.

National Alliance for the Mentally Ill
Phone: 1-800-950-NAMI (6264)

National Depressive and Manic Depressive Association
730 North Franklin Street, Suite 501, Chicago, IL 60610
Phone: 1-800-826-DMDA (3632)
Web site: http://www.ndmda.org/

National Mental Health Association
1021 Prince Street Alexandria, VA 22314-2971
Phone: 1-800-969-NMHA (6642)

American Psychological Association (APA) Consumer Help Center
Phone: 1-800-964-2000
Web site: http://helping.apa.org

PREGNANCY, INFERTILITY, AND HYPOTHYROIDISM

Taking Charge of Your Fertility, The Definitive Guide to Natural Birth Control and Pregnancy Achievement
Toni Wechsler, M.P.H.
   I consider this book the bible for understanding your menstrual cycle,

fertility, and the hormonal fluctuations each woman experiences monthly and throughout her life. This is the book we all *should* have been handed before we had our first periods.

Sher-Brody Institute for Reproductive Medicine (SBI), Geoffrey Sher, M.D.
Las Vegas, Nevada, and San Diego and La Jolla, California
Phone: 702-892-9696

Dr. Sher is a pioneer in the field of infertility in the United States and author of *In Vitro Fertilization, The A.R.T. of Making Babies*. He has expertise in working with heparin and IVIG treatments for infertility in patients with antithyroid antibodies.

WEB SITES:

- Infertility at About.com—http://infertility.about.com—An excellent starting point with articles and hundreds of links to the Web's best infertility information
- Pregnancy at About.com—http://pregnancy.about.com—My favorite pregnancy Web site

GENERAL CONVENTIONAL HEALTH INFORMATION—CENTRAL WEB SITES

Intellihealth—http://www.intellihealth.com
High-quality, overall medical site sponsored by Johns Hopkins.

Mayo Health O@sis—http://www.mayohealth.org
High-quality, overall medical/health site sponsored by the Mayo Clinic.

Thrive Online—http://www.thriveonline.com
Key consumer-oriented health site featuring diet, sports, medical, and fitness information.

OnHealth—http://www.onhealth.com/
Well-organized, informative general medical site, including conventional and alternative information, and good multimedia options as well.

Sympatico HealthyWay—http://www.nt.sympatico.ca/healthyway
Top-notch Canadian site offering medical information, community, and support on a variety of conditions.

About.com Health—http://home.about.com/health
Collection of personal expert guide-managed sites on a variety of health topics and medical conditions.

Dr. Koop's Community—http://www.drkoop.com
Good community-oriented conventional medical site founded by the former Surgeon General C. Everett Koop.

***New York Times*: Women's Health—http://www.nytimes.com/specials/women/whome/index.html**
Special section at the *New York Times'* Web site that covers health issues for women.

Mediconsult—http://www.mediconsult.com/
Comprehensive conventional medical resource site.

America's Health Network—http://www.ahn.com/
Good depth of conventional consumer-directed information, many interactive tools, and decent alternative medicine coverage.

Broadcast.com/Health—http://www.broadcast.com/SpecialInterest/healthmedical/
Featuring broadcast-on-demand of a variety of top-quality popular audio and video programs on health.

HEALTH/MEDICAL NEWS WEB SITES

Reuter's Health—http://www.reutershealth.com
News bureau for key consumer and medical stories. Reviewing and reading current consumer health news stories is free.

***New York Times'* Your Health Daily—http://yourhealthdaily.com**
Excellent archive of key health-related news stories.

MEDICAL RESEARCH WEB SITES

National Library of Medicine's PubMed—http://www.ncbi.nlm.nih.gov/ PubMed
This is the Web's premier medical research source, offering an easy searchable database of abstracts and journal references from major medical journals for more than 30 years.

Medscape—http://www.medscape.com
While primarily for health professionals, Medscape offers in-depth articles that explore the medical aspects of various issues, usually written in English consumers can understand.

Journal of the American Medical Association (JAMA)—
http://www.ama-assn.org/public/journals/jama/jamahome.htm
Key medical journal in the U.S.

*New England Journal of Medicine (NEJM)—***http://www.nejm.org**
Key medical journal in the U.S.

*British Medical Journal —***http://www.bmj.com**
Key medical journal in the U.K., features full text of many articles. Extensive coverage of hypothyroidism.

RADIO AND TELEVISION PROGRAMS ON HEALTH

Some of the key television and radio programs offering excellent coverage of conventional and alternative health issues include:

Discovery Health cable programming offers 24 hours a day of varied health-related programming. For more information, see http://www.discoveryhealth.com

Kaledioscope cable and online television offers original health programming in a range of subject areas, including a Hemative medicine. For more information, see http://www.ktv-i.cm

Jones Cable's Knowledge TV features some of television's best health programs, including: "Alternative Medicine," and "RxTV," among others. For more information, see: http://www.jec.edu/ktv/heal/index.html

Gary Null's syndicated radio show is a fresh look at alternative approaches to health. Gary also does periodic specials on public television. For more information, see: http://www.garynull.com

Zorba Paster, M.D., and Tom Clark have an excellent public radio program covering health issues. For more information, see: http://www.wpr.org/zorba

Dr. Bruce Hedendal's "Alternatives to Health" radio program goes beyond the conventional to focus on alternative healthcare options. For more information, see: http://www.broadcast.com/shows/wcma/altmed

Cable's Lifetime Network program "New Attitudes" features well-produced, informative health updates of interest to women.

HEALTH MAGAZINES AND NEWSLETTERS

Some of the best health magazines and newsletters for conventional and alternative health news include:

- Dr. Andrew Weil's *Self-Healing* newsletter
- *Alternative Medicine* magazine
- *Prevention* magazine
- *Dr. Julian Whittaker's Newsletter*
- *Townsend Letter*
- *Health* magazine
- *Natural Health*
- *Men's Health*

MUST-READ BOOKS AND
RESOURCES FOR WOMEN

Since women make up the large majority of people with hypothyroidism, I've included this category. In addition to Toni Wechsler's book *Taking Charge of Your Fertility*, mentioned earlier, these are the books I have on my bookshelf, and refer to again and again in investigating my own health issues, and in helping others know where to turn next in their searches for wellness.

Screaming to be Heard: Hormonal Connections
Women Suspect . . . and Doctors Ignore
Elizabeth Lee Vliet, M.D.

I believe every woman should read this book. Dr. Vliet is a pioneer in women's health issues, and understands that our hormones are what differentiate us from men and make us more susceptible to many diseases, ailments, and symptoms. Dr. Vliet is also a firm believer in focusing on "dealing with patients, not lab values" when it comes to thyroid disease treatment.

Listening to Your Hormones
Gillian Ford

This incredibly practical book explores the key impact hormones have on women's health and well-being, and focuses on working with doctors and hormone treatments to achieve greater wellness.

KEY WOMEN'S HORMONAL SPECIALISTS

HER Place®
Tucson, Arizona
Dallas-Ft. Worth, Texas (near DFW airport)
Phone: 817-355-8008
Web site: http://www.herplace.com

These are the women's health resource centers founded by Elizabeth Lee Vliet, M.D., author of *Screaming to be Heard: Hormonal Connections Women Suspect . . . and Doctors Ignore*. HER Place® handles in-person and consultations regarding a variety of women's hormonal health issues.

Center for Hormonal Health
South Placer Business Park
1830 Sierra Gardens Drive, #10, Roseville, CA 95661
Phone: 916-772-1681 Fax: 916-772-1683
Web site: http://www.hormonesonline.com/

Gillian Ford, Director of this Center, is the author of *Listening to Your Hormones*. Handles in-person or phone consults, and offers treatment of a wide range of hormonal disorders, including thyroid, chronic fatigue, fibromyalgia, and appropriate referral for specialist care.

Please note: If you have new resources you'd like to recommend for future updates, or if you know of updates to the information in this section, please drop me a line by email mshomon@thyroid-info.com, or regular mail, at P.O. Box 0385, Palm Harbor, FL 34682.

Alt.support.thyroid: Internet-based newsgroup for patients interested in sharing support and information about thyroid disease.

Amiodarone: A heart drug that contains iodine and can trigger thyroid problems.

Antidepressant: A medication used to treat depression.

Antiperoxidase (antimicrosomal) antibody: An antibody against peroxidase, which is a protein within the thyroid.

Antithyroid antibodies (ATA): Antibodies directed against the thyroid gland.

Antithyroid drugs: Medications that slow or stop the thyroid gland's ability to produce and synthesize thyroid hormone.

Armour Thyroid: Brand name for a nonsynthetic thyroid hormone replacement drug produced using the desiccated thyroid gland of pigs.

ATA: *See* Antithyroid antibodies

Autoimmune: Refers to a condition in which the immune system reacts against one's own tissues or organs, causing disease.

Basal body temperature: Body temperature taken immediately after waking, before any movement.

Bioequivalent: Term used to refer to a drug that has the same strength and similar availability to the body and organs when provided in the same dosage and form as another drug.

Bladderwrack: An herb that contains iodine.

Bugleweed: An herb that contains iodine.

Carbohydrate: Compounds within foods that include monosaccharides (simple sugars) like glucose, and polysaccharides (complex sugars, complex carbohydrates) like starch or cellulose.

Carpal tunnel syndrome (CTS): A condition in which compression of the median nerve in the wrist causes weakness, numbness, and pain in the hand, wrist, or fingers.

CFS: *See* Chronic Fatigue Syndrome

Chernobyl: Ukrainian site of the 1986 nuclear accident that released radiation throughout the former Soviet Union and Europe.

Chronic Fatigue Syndrome (CFS): An illness of undetermined cause that is often characterized by unexplained fatigue, weakness, muscle pain, and swollen lymph nodes.

Cold nodule: A nonfunctioning thyroid nodule/lump that does not concentrate radioactive isotopes in a thyroid scan and may be indicative of malignancy.

Congenital hypothyroidism: Hypothyroidism at or before birth, due to missing or defective thyroid gland, or dysfunction of thyroid hormone secretion and processing.

CTS: *See* Carpal tunnel syndrome

Cytomel: Brand name of liothyronine (synthetic triiodothyronine) drug sold in the U.S. and Canada.

D.O.: Doctor of Osteopathy.

Desiccated thyroid: Term used to refer to nonsynthetic thyroid hormone replacement drug produced using the thyroid gland of pigs.

Eltroxin: Canadian brand of levothyroxine.

Endocrine disruptors: Chemicals in the environment that have the ability to mimic hormones or disrupt the endocrine glands.

Endocrine glands: Glands that secrete hormonal and metabolic substances inside the body.

Endocrinologist: A doctor who specializes in treating patients with endocrine problems, including thyroid disease.

Epstein-Barr virus: A virus in the herpes family that causes infectious mononucleosis.

Estrogen: The generic term for the various female sex hormones.

Euthyroid: Refers to the condition in which the thyroid-stimulating hormone (TSH) test values are in the normal range, and the thyroid is neither hyperthyroid nor hypothyroid by test standards.

Exophthalmos: An abnormal protrusion of the eyeball from the eye socket (orbit), which can be associated with Graves' disease.

Fallout: Airborne radioactive material that falls to the ground after a nuclear accident and contaminates food and water supplies, creating potential health dangers.

Fibromyalgia: A condition characterized by pain in muscles, sleep disturbance, stiffness, and fatigue.

Follicular cancer: Second most common form of thyroid cancer.

Gland: A soft body made up of a large number of vessels that produce, store, and release—or "secrete"—some substance, often hormones.

Goiter: An enlargement of the thyroid. A goiter can be either diffuse, meaning that it is generally enlarged, or it can be nodular, asymmetrically enlarged.

Goitrogen: Referring to a substance or product that may cause thyroid enlargement and formation of a goiter.

Graves' disease: Named after Dr. Robert Graves, this is an autoimmune form of hyperthyroidism.

Graves' ophthalmopathy: An autoimmune disease, more common in Graves' disease patients, that affects the eyes.

Hashimoto's disease/thyroiditis: An autoimmune inflammation of the thyroid gland, named for Dr. Hashimoto. Can result in a goiter and often causes hypothyroidism.

HMO: Health Maintenance Organization.

Hormones: Internal secretions carried in the blood to various organs.

Hot nodule: A lump or mass on or in the thyroid gland that is often associated with hyperthyroidism.

Hyperinsulinemia: The condition in which the body produces increasing amounts of insulin in order to maintain normal blood sugar levels, causing insulin to remain in the bloodstream in higher concentrations.

Hyperthyroidism: Excess production of thyroid hormone, due to abnormal thyroid gland function, nodules, or excessive thyroid hormone replacement.

Hypothalamus: A part of the brain that has a key role in endocrine function. It conducts thyroid hormone conversion.

Hypothermia: The condition of low body temperature.

Hypothyroidism: Insufficient production of thyroid hormone due to abnormal thyroid gland function, absence of all or part of the thyroid gland, or insufficient thyroid hormone replacement.

Insulin: Hormone released by the pancreas that helps process sugar in the blood.

Iodine: An element—found in seafood and added to supplements and salt—that is the most essential component for the body's ability to manufacture thyroid hormone.

Iodine-131: A form of iodine that, when released in sufficient quantities due to nuclear accidents or nuclear releases, can cause thyroid disease. Also used as a form of treatment for some overactive thyroid conditions.

Isthmus: The area connecting the two lobes of the thyroid gland.

Kelp: A form of seaweed containing high amounts of iodine.

Levothroid: A brand of synthetic thyroxine (levothyroxine) sold in the U.S.

Levothyroxine, Levothyroxine sodium: The generic name for synthetic thyroxine, also known as T4, a thyroid hormone replacement drug. Brand names in the U.S. and Canada include Synthroid, Levothroid, Levoxyl, Eltroxin, and PMS-Levothyroxine.

Levoxyl: A brand of levothyroxine sold in the U.S.

Libido: Sex drive.

Liothyronine: The generic name for the drug that is a synthetic version of triiodothyronine, T3.

Liotrix: A synthetic drug combining levothyroxine and liothyronine (synthetic T4 plus synthetic T3).

Lithium: A drug used to treat manic depression known to cause thyroid disease in some patients.

Lobes: A term that refers to the two sides of the thyroid gland.

Medullary cancer: The third most common form of thyroid cancer involving a specialized thyroid cell—the C cell—that manufactures calcitonin.

Metabolism: The process by which oxygen and calories are converted to energy for use by cells and organs.

Methimazole: An antithyroid medication used to treat hyperthyroidism.

Mitral Valve Prolapse (MVP): A heart condition in which improper closure of one of the heart valves creates slight regurgitation, often accompanied by an audible "murmur."

Mono-deiodination: The conversion process by which one iodine molecule is removed from thyroxine (T4) converting it to triiodothyronine (T3), also known as T4 to T3 conversion.

Mononucleosis: A condition of the lymph glands caused by infection with Epstein-Barr virus.

Multinodular goiter: A condition in which the thyroid is enlarged and has two or more nodules.

Myxedema: A condition characterized by swelling of skin and other tissues, particularly with puffiness around the eyes and cheeks, caused by hypothyroidism.

Myxedemic coma: Severe myxedemia, often accompanied with hypothermia, resulting in unconsciousness.

Natural thyroid: Nonsynthetic thyroid hormone replacement drug produced using the desiccated thyroid gland of pigs.

Naturethroid: Brand name for a hypo-allergenic natural thyroid hormone replacement drug produced using the desiccated thyroid gland of pigs, sold in the U.S.

Naturopathy: Holistic medical practice based on a balance of physical, emotional, mental, and spiritual aspects, and the body's innate ability to heal itself.

Nodular goiter: An enlargement of the thyroid gland characterized by one or more nodules.

Nodule: A lump or abnormal growth of tissue on or within the thyroid.

Osteopathy: A form of medicine that, in addition to medication and nutrition, relies on osteopathic manipulation, the process of working with the imbalances and misalignment in the body's musculoskeletal system as a way to treat illness.

Osteoporosis: A condition in which calcium lost from the bones makes bones brittle and more easily broken. Most common in older women and men.

Palpitation: The condition of feeling the heart beating, whether due to rapid heartbeat, irregular or missed beats, or just strong, forceful beating.

Papillary cancer: The most common form of thyroid cancer, often caused by radiation exposure.

Parathyroid glands: Small, paired endocrine glands located behind the thyroid that secrete parathyroid hormone and control calcium and bone metabolism.

Perchlorate: A chemical used in the manufacture of rockets and fireworks that, when contaminating the water supply, can adversely affect the thyroid.

Phytoestrogen: A plant product that acts like an estrogen and has an effect on the endocrine system, e.g., soy.

Pituitary gland: A small, peanut-sized gland located behind the eyes at the base of the brain. It secretes hormones that control other endocrine glands, and specifically, secretes thyroid-stimulating hormone.

PMS-Levothyroxine: The Canadian brand of levothyroxine.

Polycystic Ovary Syndrome (PCOS): A syndrome characterized by heavy or absent periods, lack of ovulation, and cysts on the ovaries.

Postpartum: Refers to the period after pregnancy.

Postpartum thyroiditis: A temporary inflammation of the thyroid, occurring after pregnancy, that can result in transient hypothyroidism.

Potassium iodide: A drug used to treat certain thyroid disorders that can also be taken after nuclear accidents to protect the thyroid from damage by blocking the gland's uptake of radio-active-iodine isotopes.

Premenstrual Syndrome (PMS): Emotional, physical, psychological, and mood-related symptoms that take place in the menstrual cycle after ovulation and just prior to menstruation.

Progesterone: A hormone produced in the corpus luteum of the ovary.

Propylthiouracil (PTU): An antithyroid medication used for hyperthyroidism that blocks thyroid cells from producing thyroid hormone.

PTU: *See* Propylthiouracil

Radioactive iodine (RAI): A radioactive form of iodine that is used to diagnose and treat thyroid problems.

Resistance to Thyroid Hormone (RTH): Insufficient cellular response to thyroid hormone that can result in hypothyroidism.

Reverse T3: A form of inactive triiodothyronine (T3) that is formed during periods of stress on the body.

Subclinical hypothyroidism: Mild hypothyroidism that does not necessarily have associated symptoms.

Suppression: The process of providing enough thyroid hormone replacement to thyroid cancer survivors to "suppress" TSH to low, or barely detectable levels, in order to prevent thyroid cancer recurrence.

Synthroid: The brand of levothyroxine sold in the U.S. and Canada.

T3: Shorthand for triiodothyronine, the more potent of the two key hormones produced by the thyroid gland. Triiodothyronine is also produced from the conversion of thyroxine (T4) in tissue and cells.

T4: Shorthand for thyroxine, the primary hormone produced by the thyroid gland.

T4 to T3 conversion: The conversion process by which one iodine molecule is removed from thyroxine (T4), converting it to triiodothyronine (T3). Also known as mono-deiodination.

Tapazole: The brand name of an antithyroid drug.

TBG: *See* Thyroid Binding Globulin

Testosterone: A male sex hormone present in both men and women.

TG: *See* Thyroglobulin

Thiocyanate: A chemical found in cigarettes and some foods that can cause thyroid dysfunction.

Thyrogen: A drug that is administered to some thyroid cancer survivors prior to diagnostic scans that allows for scanning without withdrawal from thyroid hormone and resulting hypothyroidism.

Thyroglobulin (TG): A protein in the thyroid gland that can be used as a marker for thyroid disease and thyroid cancer.

Thyroid Binding Globulin (TBG): A protein in the bloodstream that binds with thyroxine.

Thyroid Eye Disease: Autoimmune-related eye condition that accompanies autoimmune thyroid disease.

Thyroid gland: Butterfly-shaped gland located in the lower part of the neck, in front of the windpipe, that secretes hormones that regulate metabolism.

Thyroid-Stimulating Hormone (TSH, Thyrotropin): A hormone produced by the pituitary gland that stimulates the thyroid gland. Measurement of the levels of this drug is considered a primary way to assess hypothyroidism and hyperthyroidism.

Thyroidectomy: The surgical removal of all or part of the thyroid gland.

Thyroiditis: An inflammation of the thyroid gland.

Thyrolar: Brand name for the synthetic drug combining levothyroxine and liothyronine (synthetic T4 plus synthetic T3).

Thyrotropin-Releasing Hormone (TRH): A hormone released by the hypothalamus that communicates with the pituitary gland and stimulates release of thyroid-stimulating hormone.

Thyrotropin-Releasing Hormone (TRH) Test: A highly sensitive test that detects abnormal thyroid function.

Thyrotropin: *See* Thyroid-Stimulating Hormone

Thyroxine (T4): The primary hormone produced by the thyroid gland.

Toxic goiter: An enlarged thyroid gland that is causing hyperthyroidism.

TRH: *See* Thyrotropin Releasing Hormone

TRH Test: A highly sensitive test that detects abnormal thyroid function.

Triiodothyronine (T3): The more potent of the two key hormones produced by the thyroid gland. Triiodothyronine is also produced from the conversion of thyroxine (T4) in tissue and cells.

TSH: *See* Thyroid Stimulating Hormone

Tyrosine: An amino acid necessary for the production of thyroid hormone.

Westhroid: The brand name for a nonsynthetic thyroid hormone replacement drug produced using the desiccated thyroid gland of pigs.

Wilson's Syndrome: Self-named syndrome identified by a former M.D., who believes that stress on the body causes chronic low body temperature and Reverse T3 production.

REFERENCES

Introduction

Bunevicius, Robertas, et al. "Effects of Thyroxine as Compared with Thyroxine plus Triiodothyronine in Patients with Hypothyroidism." *New England Journal of Medicine.* 340 (1999):424–429, 469–470.

Kellman, Rafael, M.D. "Energizing Chronic Fatigue." *Alternative Medicine* September 1997.

Chapter 2

American Association of Clinical Endocrinologists. Web site information. http://www.aace.com

American Medical Women's Association. "Facts about thyroid disease." Health Topics, http://www.amwa-doc.org/healthtopics/thyroid.html#Overview

American Thyroid Association. "Thyroid Disease in the Elderly." [Online patient brochure] http://www.thyroid.org/patient/brochur2.htm

Arizona Republic. "Pollutant Likely Migrated Via Canal." 27 August 1998.

"Ask Dr. Weil." *Bulletin Boards.* http://www.drweil.com

Atcheson, Steven G., M.D. "Concurrent Medical Disease in Work-Related Carpal Tunnel Syndrome." *Archives of Internal Medicine,* July 27, 1998, et. al. 158(1998):1506–1512. http://www.ama-assn.org/sci-pubs/journals/archive/inte/vol_158/no_14/ioi70670.htm

Brauman, A., et al. "Prevalence of mitral valve prolapse in chronic lymphocytic thyroiditis and nongoitrous hypothyroidism." *Cardiology* 75(4)(1998): 269–73.

Fukata, S., et. al. "Relationship between cigarette smoking and hypothyroidism in patients with Hashimoto's thyroiditis." *J Endocrinol Invest.* 19(9) (Oct 1996):607–12.

"GlandCentral Campaign." Website information. http://www.glandcentral.com

Greene, Loren Wissner, M.D., F.A.C.P., F.A.C.E. "The Thyroid and Reproductive System, Disorders of Menstruation, Fertility and Pregnancy." *The Bridge.* [Thyroid Foundation of America newsletter] 10(1). http://www.clark.net/pub/tfa/bridge/bridge.vol10.no1.html

Hanford Health Information Network. *An Overview of Hanford Health and Radiation Effects.* http://www.doh.wa.gov/hanford/publications/overview/overview.html

Journal of Clinical Endocrinology and Metabolism. 82(1997):2455–2457.

Las Vegas Review-Journal. "Rocket fuel chemical found in Arizona water." 28 August 1998.

National Cancer Institute. "Exposure of The American People To I-131 From Nevada Atmospheric Bomb Tests." *Technical Summary TS.5. Estimation of the Thyroid Doses from U-131.* (1997). http://rex.nci.nih.gov/massmedia/reporttofc.html

Newton, Gail, D., Ph.D., R.Ph., "Hasimoto's Thyroiditis." *U.S. Pharmacist: The Journal for Pharmacists' Education* (December 1998).

Obstetrics and Gynecology. 90(1997):364–369.

Sehnert, K.W., et al. "Basal metabolic temperature vs. laboratory assessment in 'posttraumatic hypothyroidism,'" *Manipulative Physiol Ther.* 19(1) (Jan 1996):6–12.

The Tennessean. Nuclear Plant Health Series, 29 September 1998.

Thyroid Foundation of America. "Childhood Head and Neck Irradiation." http://www.clark.net/pub/tfa/brochure/brochure-irrad.html

University of California at Davis. *MTBE Research.* http://tsrtp.ucdavis.edu/mtbe/

UPI. "Testing urged for thousands of chemicals." 5 October 1998.

Utiger, Robert D., M.D. "Cigarette Smoking and the Thyroid." *New England Journal of Medicine.* 333(15) (12 October 1995).

Waylonis, G.W., and W. Heck. "Fibromyalgia syndrome. New associations." *J Phys Med Rehabil.* 71(6) (Dec 1992):343–8.

Wolf, J. "Perchlorate and the thyroid gland." *Pharmacol Rev.* 50(1) (Mar 1998):89–105.

Buffalo News. "Researcher Warns of Potential Global Health Crisis." 7 October 1998.

Chapter 3

Adlin, Victor, M.D. "Subclinical Hypothyroidism: Deciding When to Treat." *American Family Physician Magazine,* 15 February 1998. [Online edition]. http://www.aafp.org/afp/980215ap/adlin.html

American Association of Clinical Endocrinologists. "Symptoms List." http://www.aace.com/pub/spec/tam98/symptoms.html

American Tinnitus Association. Website. http://www.ata.org

Barnes, Broda, O.M.D., and Lawrence Galton. *Hypothyroidism: The Unsuspected Illness.* New York: Harper & Row, 1976.

Berkow, Robert, M.D. *The Merck Manual of Diagnosis and Therapy.* New Jersey: Merck & Company, 1999.

Bhatia P.L., Gupta O.P., Agrawal M.K., Mishr S.K. "Audiological and vestibular function tests in hypothyroidism." *Laryngoscope* 87(12) (Dec 1977):2082–9.

Greene, Loren Wissner M.D., F.A.C.P., F.A.C.E., "The Thyroid and Reproductive System, Disorders of Menstruation, Fertility and Pregnancy." *The Bridge* [Thyroid Foundation of America newsletter] 10(1). http://www.clark.net/pub/tfa/bridge/bridge.vol10.no1.html

Journal of Clinical Endocrinology and Metabolism. 82 (August 1997):2455–57

Lasser, R. A., Baldessarini, R. J. "Thyroid hormones in depressive disorders: a reappraisal of clinical utility." *Harv Rev Psychiatry* 4(6) (Mar–Apr 1997):291–305.

Laumann, Edward O., Ph.D., et al. "Sexual Dysfunction in the United States, Prevalence and Predictors." *Journal of the American Medical Association* 281(6) (10 February 1999).

National Institutes of Health, National Heart, Lung, and Blood Institute. "Facts About High Blood Pressure." http://www.nih.gov/health/htp-hbp/3.htm

National Sleep Foundation. Website. http://www.sleepfoundation.org

Obstetrics and Gynecology 90(1997):364–69.

Obstetrics and Gynecology 92(1998):206–11.

"Prescribing Trends in Psychotropic Medications." *Journal of the American Medical Association* 279(7) (18 February 1998).

Thyroid Foundation of America. *Hypothyroidism.* Thyroid Topics Brochures, 1995 [online version]. http://www.clark.net/pub/tfa/brochure/brochure-hypo.html

Vliet, Elizabeth Lee, M.D. *Screaming to Be Heard : Hormonal Connections Women Suspect . . . and Doctors Ignore.* New York: M Evans & Co., 1995.

Wilson's Syndrome Foundation. Web site. http://www.wilssonssyndrone.com

Chapter 4

Adlin, Victor, M.D. "Subclinical Hypothyroidism: Deciding When to Treat." *American Family Physician Magazine,* 15 February 1998. [Online edition]. http://www.aafp.org/afp/980215ap/adlin.html

Danforth, E. Jr; Burger, A. "The role of thyroid hormones in the control of energy expenditure." *Clinics in Endocrinology and Metabolism* 13 (3) (Nov 1984):581–95.

Dzurec, L. C. "Experiences of fatigue and depression before and after low-dose 1-thyroxine supplementation in essentially euthyroid individuals." *Research in Nursing and Health* 20 (5) (Oct 1997):389–98.

Fowler, P. B.; McIvor, J.; Sykes, L.; Macrae, K.D. "The effect of long-term thyroxine on bone mineral density and serum cholesterol." *Journal of the Royal College of Physicians of London.* 30 (6) (1996):527–32.

Grant, D. J.; McMurdo, M. E.; Mole, P. A.; Paterson, C. R.; Davies, R. R. "Suppressed TSH levels secondary to thyroxine replacement therapy are not associated with osteoporosis." *Clinical Endocrinology.* 39 (5) (Nov 1993):529–33.

Kellman, Rafael, M.D. "Energizing Chronic Fatigue." *Alternative Medicine.* Issue 19 (September 1997).

Leviton, Richard. "Reviving the Thyroid." *Alternative Medicine Digest.* Issue 22 (February/March 1998).

Ross, D. S. "Hyperthyroidism, thyroid hormone therapy, and bone." *Thyroid* 4 (3) (Fall 1994): 319–26.

Singh, A.; Dantas, Z. N.; Stone, S. C.; Asch, R. H. "Presence of thyroid antibodies in early reproductive failure: biochemical versus clinical pregnancies." *Fertility and Sterility* 63 (2) (Feb 1995):277–81.

Weil, Andrew, M.D. *Natural Health, Natural Medicine.* New York: Houghton Mifflin Co., 1990.

"The Many Faces of Fatigue." *U.S. Pharmacist,* 23(12) (1998).

"Physicians: Hardest hit by healthcare reform." *Health Care Review,* September 1996.

Weetman, A. P. "Clinical review: Fortnightly review: Hypothyroidism: screening and subclinical disease." *British Medical Journal.* 314 (19 April 1997):1175.

Chapter 5

Konno, N., et al. "Seasonal variation of serum thyrotropin concentration and thyrotropin response to thyrotropin-releasing hormone in patients with primary hypothyroidism on constant replacement dosage of thyroxine." *Journal of Clinical Endocrinology and Metabolism* 54 (6) (1982):1118–24.

Lakshmy, R., et al. "Iodine metabolism in response to goitrogen induced altered thyroid status under conditions of moderate and high intake of iodine." *Hormone and Metabolic Research* 27 (10) (Oct 1995):450–4.

Maes, M., et al. "Components of biological variation, including seasonality, in blood concentrations of TSH, TT3, FT4, PRL, cortisol and testosterone in healthy volunteers." *Clinical Endocrinology* 46 (5) (May 1997):587–98.

McCowen, K. C., et al. "Elevated serum thyrotropin in thyroxine-treated patients with hypothyroidism given sertraline." *New England Journal of Medicine* 2;337(14) (Oct 1997):1010–11.

Nicolau, G. Y., et. al. "Chronobiology of pituitary-thyroid functions." *Romanian Journal of Endocrinology* 30 (3-4) (1992):125–48.

Nishi, I., et al. "Intra-individual and seasonal variations of thyroid function tests in healthy subjects." *Rinsho Byori. Japanese Journal of Clinical Pathology.* 44 (2) (1996):159–62.

Reed, H. L. "Circannual changes in thyroid hormone physiology: the role of cold environmental temperatures." *Arctic Medical Research* 54 Suppl 2 (1995):9–15.

Schneyer, Christine R., M.D. "Letters—March 11, 1998 Calcium Carbonate and Reduction of Levothyroxine Efficacy." *Journal of the American Medical Association* 279 (11 March 1998):750.

Chapter 6

Capen, C. C. "TI: Mechanistic data and risk assessment of selected toxic end points of the thyroid gland." *Toxicologic Pathology* 25 (1) (Jan–Feb 1997):39–48.

Centers for Disease Control. *CDC's Diabetes and Public Health Resource.* http://www.cdc.gov/diabetes/

De Rosa, G., et al. "A slightly suppressive dose of L-thyroxine does not affect bone turnover and bone mineral density in pre- and postmenopausal women with nontoxic goitre." *Hormone Metabolic Research.* Italy 27(11) (Nov 1995):503–7.

Elfstrom, David. "How to Talk to Doctors." http://www.sunnybrook.utoronto. ca/~elfstrom/arthritis/articles/appointments.html

Florkowski, C. M., et al. "Bone mineral density in patients receiving suppressive doses of thyroxine for thyroid carcinoma." *New Zealand Medical Journal* 106(966) (Oct 1993):443–44.

Grant, D. J., et al. "Suppressed TSH levels secondary to thyroxine replacement therapy are not associated with osteoporosis." *Clinical Endocrinology* (Oxford) 39(5) (Nov 1993):529–33.

College of Agriculture and Life Sciences, Cornell University, Comstock Hall, Ithaca, New York 14853-0901; Hawaii Department of Agriculture, Division of Plant Industry, Honolulu, Hawaii 96814.

Ross, Douglas S., M.D. "Ask the Doctor." *The Bridge.* 13(2) (Summer 1998).

Weetman, A. P. "Clinical review: Fortnightly review: Hypothyroidism: screening and subclinical disease." *British Medical Journal.* 314 (19 April 1997):1175.

Chapter 7

Balch, James F., M.D., and Phyllis Balch. *Prescription for Nutritional Healing: A Practical A-Z Reference to Drug-Free Remedies Using Vitamins, Minerals, Herbs & Food Supplements.* Avery, Garden City Park, NY 1996.

Berger, M. M., et al. "Relations between the selenium status and the low T3 syndrome after major trauma" *Intensive Care Medicine* 22 (6) (Jun 1996):575–81.

"Clinical study of yoga techniques in university students with asthma: a controlled study." *Allergy Asthma Proc.* 19(1): (Jan–Feb 1998)3–9.

Hollowell, J.G., et al. "Iodine nutrition in the United States. Trends and public health implications: iodine excretion data from National Health and Nutrition Examination Surveys I and III (1971–1974 and 1988–1994)." *J Clin Endocrinol Metab* 83(10) (Oct 1998):3401–8.

Hotz, C. S., et al. "Dietary Iodine and selenium interact to affect thyroid hormone metabolism of rats." *Journal of Nutrition* 127 (6) (Jun 1997):1214–8.

Kellman, Rafael, M.D. "Energizing Chronic Fatigue." *Alternative Medicine*, September 1997.

Landis, Robyn. *Herbal Defense.* New York: Warner Books, 1997.

Langer, Stephen E., M.D. *Solved: The Riddle of Illness.* New York: Keats, 1995.

Leviton, Richard. "Reviving the Thyroid." *Alternative Medicine.* Issue 22 (February/March 1998).

National Institutes of Health. *Complementary and Alternative Medicine Newsletter* V(1) (Jan 1998).

"P300 amplitude and antidepressant response to Sudarshan Kriya Yoga." *Journal of Affective Disorders.* 50(1) (Jul 1998):45–8.

"Trends in Alternative Medicine Use in the United States, 1990–1997 Results of a Follow-up National Survey." *Journal of the American Medical Association.* 280(18) (1998).

Tripathi, Yamini B., et al. "Thyroid Stimulating Action of Z-Guggulsterone Obtained from Commiphora mukul." *Planta Medica,* (1) (Feb 1984):78–80.

Xu, M., et al. "Effect of Chinese herbs on the circadian rhythm of body temperature." *Chung-Kuo Chung Yao Tsa Chih China Journal of Chinese Materia Medica* 4 (21 April 1996):247–49.

"Yoga-Based Intervention for Carpal Tunnel Syndrome." *Journal of the American Medical Association.* 281 (11 November 1998): 2087.

Zha, L. L. "Relation of hypothyroidism and deficiency of kidney yang." *Chung-Kuo Chung Yao Tsa Chih China Journal of Chinese Materia Medica.* 13 (4) (1993):202–4.

Zhang, J. Q. "Effects of yin-tonics and yang-tonics on serum thyroid hormone levels." *Chung-Kuo Chung Yao Tsa Chih China Journal of Chinese Materia Medica* II(2) (February 1991).

Chapter 8

Aarflot, T. "Association between chronic widespread musculoskeletal complaints and thyroid autoimmunity. Results from a community survey." *Scandinavian Journal of Primary Health Care* 14 (2) (1996):111–5.

Anisman, H., et al. "Neuroimmune mechanisms in health and disease." *Canadian Medical Association Journal* 155(8) (Oct 1998):1075–82.

Bell, David S. *The Doctor's Guide to Chronic Fatigue Syndrome: Understanding, Treating, and Living with CFIDS.* Cambridge, MA: Perseus Books, 1995.

Blanchard, Kenneth, M.D. Telephone interviews with Mary Shomon, October 1998.

Boschert, Sherry. "T3 Plus T4 'Unproven' for Hypothyroidism," *Internal Medicine News,* 1 May 1999.

Bunevicius, Robertas; et. al. "Effects of Thyroxine as Compared with Thyroxine plus Triiodothyronine in Patients with Hypothyroidism." *New England Journal of Medicine* 340(1999):424–429, 469–470.

"Chronic fatigue syndrome: influence of histamine, hormones and electrolytes." *Medical Hypotheses.* 1993

Hilgers, A. "Chronic fatigue syndrome: immune dysfunction, role of pathogens and toxic agents and neurological and cardiac changes." *Wien Med Wochenschr.* 144(16) (1994):399–406.

Konstantinov, K., et al. "Autoantibodies to nuclear envelope antigens in chronic fatigue syndrome." *Journal of Clinical Investigation.* 98(8) (Oct 15 1996):1888–96.

Leslie, P. J., and Toft, A. D. "The replacement therapy problem in hypothyroidism." *Baillieres Clinical Endocrinology and Metabolism* 2 (3) (Aug 1998):653–69.

Lowe, John C., D.C. Telephone and email interviews with Mary Shomon, October 1998.

Lowe, John C., et al. "Mutations in the c-erbA beta 1 gene: do they underlie euthyroid fibromyalgia?" *Medical Hypotheses* 48 (2) (1997):125–35.

Lowe, John C. "Thyroid status of 38 fibromyalgia patients: Implications for the etiology of fibromyalgia." *Clinical Bulletin of Myofascial Therapy* 2 (1997): 47–64.

Toft, Anthony D., M.D. "Thyroid Hormone Replacement—One Hormone or Two?" *New England Journal of Medicine.* 340(6) (1999).

Chapter 9

American Diabetes Association. Web site. http://www.diabetes.org

Arnot, Robert, M.D. *Dr. Bob Arnot's Revolutionary Weight Control Program.* Boston: Little Brown & Co., 1998.

Aronne, Louis J., M.D. *Weigh Less, Live Longer : Dr. Lou Aronne's 'Getting Healthy' Plan for Permanent Weight Control.* New York: John Wiley & Sons, 1996.

Ezrin, Calvin, M.D. *The Type II Diabetes Diet Book.* Los Angeles: Lowell House Publishers, 1999.

Siafakas, N. M., et al. "Respiratory muscle strength in hypothyroidism." *Chest* 102(1) (Jul 1992):189–94.

Thyroid Foundation of America. "Is Your Thyroid Making You Fat." Boston, Massachusetts: 25 June 1996.

Chapter 10

Hsiung, Robert, M.D. "Dr. Bob's Psychopharmcology Tips." http://uhs.bsd.uchicago.edu/dr-bob/tips/tips.html

McGaffee, J., et al. "Psychiatric presentations of hypothyroidism." *American Family Physician.* 23 (5) (May 1981):129–33.

National Institute of Mental Health. Web site. http://www.nimh.nih.gov

Nemeroff, Charles B. "The Neurobiology of Depression." *Scientific American.* (June 1998). http://www.sciam.com/1998/0698issue/0698nemeroff.html

Pies, Ron M.D. "The Diagnosis and Treatment of Subclinical Hypothyroid States in Depressed Patients." *General Hospital Psychiatry.* 19 (1997):344–54.

Pies, Ron M.D. "Mental Health Infosource." *Psychiatric Times.* http://www.mhsource.com/expert/exp1092396h.html

Chapter 11

Glinoer, D., et al. "Risk of subclinical hypothyroidism in pregnant women with asymptomatic autoimmune thyroid disorders." *Journal of Clinical Endocrinology and Metabolism* 79 (1) (July 1994):197–204.

Haddow, James E., et al. "Maternal Thyroid Deficiency during Pregnancy and Subsequent Neuropsychological Development of the Child," *The New England Journal of Medicine* 341(8) (Aug 1999).

Iijima, Takashi. *Obstetrics and Gynecology.* 90 (Sept 1997):364–69.

Mandel, Susan J. "Thyroiditis After Pregnancy Loss." *Journal of Clinical Endocrinology and Metabolism* 82(8) (Aug 1997):2455–57.

Obstetrics & Gynecology. 92(2) (Aug 1998):206–211.

Tamaki H., et. al. "Thyroxine requirement during pregnancy for replacement therapy of hypothyroidism." *Obstetrics and Gynecology.* 76 (2) (Aug 1990):230–3.

Weschler, Toni. *Taking Charge of Your Fertility: The Definitive Guide to Natural Birth Control and Pregnancy Achievement.* New York: HarperPerennial, 1995.

Chapter 12

Cherkes, Kelly. Email and telephone interviews with Mary Shomon, October 1998.

Chapter 13

Thyrogen Product Information. Genzyme Web site. http://www.genzyme.com

Epilogue

Burman, K. D., et al. "A radioimmunoassay for 3,3',5'-L-triiodothyronine (reverse T3): assessment of thyroid gland content and serum measurements in conditions of normal and altered thyroidal economy and following administration of thyrotropin releasing hormone (TRH) and thyrotropin (TSH)." *Journal of Clinical Endocrinology and Metabolism.* 44 (4) (Apr 1977):660–72.

Canaris, G. J., Manowitz, N., Mayor, G., and Ridgway, E. C. "Prevalence of Abnormal Lipid Abnormalities and Symptoms of Thyroid Disease in a Large Observational Cohort," Paper presented to the 70th Annual Meeting of the American Thyroid Association, Sunday, 19 October 1997.

Cassidy, A., et al. "Biological effects of a diet of soy protein rich in isoflavones on the menstrual cycle of premenopausal women." *Am J Clin Nutr.* 60: (1994) 333-340.

Chapin, et. al. "Endocrine modulation of reproduction." *Fund Appl Tox.* 29: 1996 1-17.

Chorazy, P. A., et al. "Persistent hypothyroidism in an infant receiving a soy formula: case report and review of the literature." *Pediatrics.* 1995 148–150.

Clarkson, T. B., et al. "Estrogenic soybean isoflavones and chronic disease. Risks and benefits." *Trends Endocrinol Metab* 6 (1995):11–16.

Colborn, Theodora, et al. *Our Stolen Future.* London: Little Brown and Company, 1996.

Cruz, et al. "Effects of infant nutrition on cholesterol synthesis rates." *Ped Res* 35 (1994):135–140.

Divi, R. L.; Doerge, D. R. "Inhibition of thyroid peroxidase by dietary flavonoids." *Chemical Research in Toxicology* 9 (1) (Jan–Feb 1996):16–23.

Divi, R. L., et al. "Anti-thyroid isoflavones from the soybean." *Biochem Pharmacol* 54(1997):1087–96.

Drane, H. M., et al. "Oestrogenic activity of soya-bean products." *Fd Cosmet.-Technol.* 18 (1980):425–27.

Fitzpatrick, Dr. Mike and Dibb, Sue. "Soya Infant Formula: the Health Concerns." *Food Commission Briefing Paper* (October 1998), London, UK.

Fontanarosa, Phil B., M.D.; Lundberg, George D., M.D. "Alternative Medicine Meets Science—Editorial." *Journal of the American Medical Association* 280(18) (Nov 1998).

Fort, P., et al. "Breast and soy-formula feeding feedings in early infancy and the prevalence of autoimmune thyroid disease in children." *J Am Coll Nutr* 9 (April 1990):164–67.

Fort, et. al. "Breast feeding and insulin-dependent diabetes mellitus in children." *J Am Coll Nutr* 5 (Feb 1986) 439–41.

Hollowell, J. G., et al. "Iodine nutrition in the United States. Trends and public health implications: iodine excretion data from National Health and Nutrition Examination Surveys I and III (1971–1974 and 1988–1994)." *J Clin Endocrinol Metab* 83(10) (Oct 1998):3401–8.

Hydovitz, J. D. "Occurrence of goiter in an infants on a soy diet." *New Eng J Med* 262 (1960): 351–53.

Infant and Dietetic Foods Association. "Phytoestrogens in Soya Infant Formula." Letter to the Food Commission, 24 September 1998.

Irvine, C.H.G., et al. "Phytoestrogens in soy-based infant foods: concentrations, daily intake, and possible biological effects." *PSEBM* 217 (1998):247–53.

Ishizuki, Y., et. al. "The effects on the thyroid gland of soybeans administered experimentally in healthy subjects." *Nippon Naibunpi gakkai Zasshi.* 67 (1991): 622–29.

Jabbar, M. A., et. al. "Abnormal thyroid function tests in infants with congenital hypothyroidism: the influence of soy-based formula." *J Am Coll Nutr.* 16 (1997): 280–82.

King, Ralph, Jr. "Judge Blocks Proposed Synthroid Pact, Criticizing the Level of Attorneys' Fees." *The Wall Street Journal,* 2 September 1998.

Knoll Pharmaceuticals. *Knoll Settles Thyroid Medication Class Action Lawsuit.* Press release, 4 August 1997.

"Levothyroxine New Drug Application Information." *Federal Register.* 62 (1997).

Murphy, P. A., et al. "Isoflavones in Soy-Based Infant Formulas." *J Agric Food Chem* 45(1997): 4635–38.

Ostrum, Janus L. "Tolerance of soy formulas with reduced phytate/phytoestrogens fed to healthy term children." *Presentation at the Second International Symposium on the Role of Soy in Preventing and Treating Chronic Disease.* Brussels, September 16-19, 1996.

Peat, Ray, Ph.D. "Thyroid: Misconceptions." *Townsend Letter for Doctors.* (November 1993).

Pinchera, A., et al. "Thyroid refractoriness in an athyreotic cretin fed soybean formula." *New Eng J Med.* 273(1965): 83–87.

Rennie, Drummond M.D. "Thyroid Storm." Editorial. *Journal of the American Medical Association.* (April 1997).

Ripp, J. A. "Soybean induced goiter." *Am J Dis Child* 102(1961): 136–39.

Rxlist.com. http://www.rxlist.com/

Ryan, P. J. "The Effects of Thyroxine Therapy on Bone Mineral Density." *Journal of Clinical Densitometry* 1(2)(1998):173–77.

Santi, R., et al. "Phytoestrogens: potential endocrine disruptors in males." *Tox Ind Health.* 14 (1998):223–237.

Setchell, K.D.R., et al. "Exposure of infants to phytoestrogens from soy-based infant formula." *Lancet.* 350 (1997):23–27.

Sheeham, D. M. "Isoflavone content of breast milk and soy formulas: benefits and risks (letter)." *Clin Chem.* 43(1997):850.

Sherrill, Robert. "A Year in Corporate Crime." *The Nation.* (1997). http://www.thenation.com:80/issue/970407/0407sher.htm

Synthroid Lawsuit Claims. Website. http://www.synthroidclaims.com

Van Wyk, et. al. "The effects of a soybean product on thyroid function in humans." *Pediatrics* 24 (1959): 752–60.

Wang, H., and Murphy, P. A. "Isoflavone content in commercial soybean foods." *J Agric Food Chem.* 42(1994): 1666–73.

Weetman, A. P. "Clinical review: Fortnightly review: Hypothyroidism: screening and subclinical disease." *British Medical Journal.* 314(19 Apr 1997):1175.

INDEX

11/21/01 = TSH = 11.88, free T4 = .7, free T3 = 2.62

2/2/02 = TSH = 4.42

considered Normal range 4.9 - 4.67
Acc to Dr. Stearn's office